THE ULTIMATE

PICKLEBALL

JOURNAL

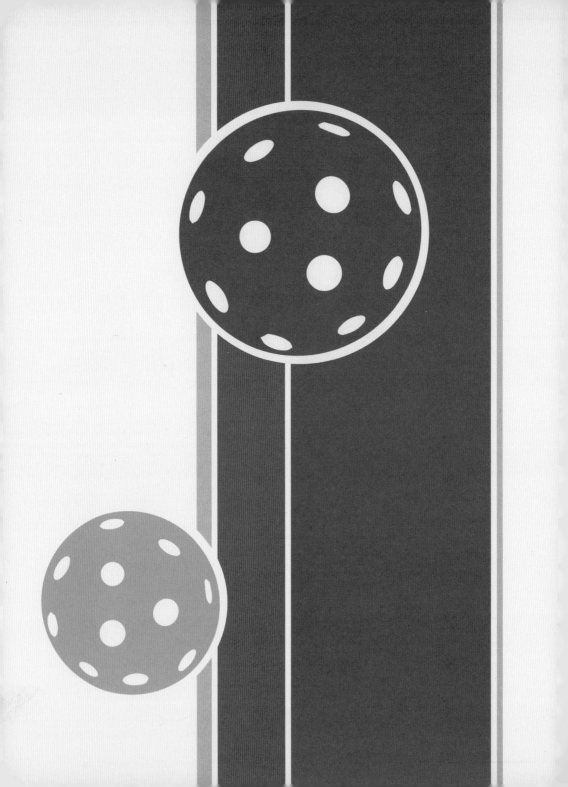

THE ULTIMATE
PICKLEBALL
JOURNAL

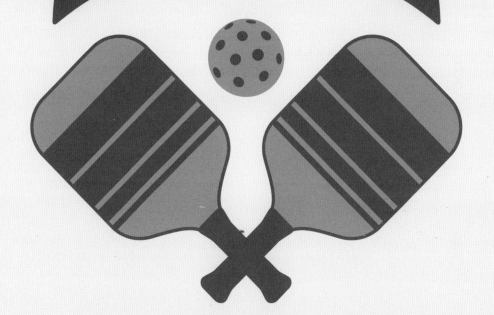

CHART YOUR PROGRESS AND RECORD YOUR GAMES!

Sydney Steinaker

Illustrated by Lucía Gómez Alcaide

ROCK
POINT

CONTENTS

INTRODUCTION

Welcome to the wonderful world of pickleball! If you've picked up this journal, then you're ready to get serious about this popular sport phenomenon.

A helpful guide for players of any skill level, this go-to game companion includes everything you need to know to get ready to play—a historic overview of the game, key pickleball lingo, game basics, must-have equipment, an insider's guide to tournament life, and tips for getting your body and mind right for game day. Once you've immersed yourself in all that is pickledom, track your athletic development with over a year's worth of journal pages featuring checklists and assessments to help improve your game.

Whatever your pickleball goals are, *The Ultimate Pickleball Journal* will help you in your journey to becoming a more well-rounded athlete and ready to take to the courts.

HOW TO USE THIS JOURNAL

Before you grab your paddles and swing, read about the rise of pickleball, learn the lingo, and determine which equipment best suits you. Review the pickleball game basics over and over until you have familiarized yourself with the moves, and practice on your own outside of any official games to start.

Once you start playing, you can track your progress at the back of this journal using monthly planners designed to build a consistent routine in your pickleball training. Note your areas of weaknesses and strengths as part of your skills assessments, record your individual games and scores, and take advantage of the goal-setting templates to further your competitive gameplay.

Good luck and let's play!

THE RISE *of* PICKLEBALL

So, what exactly is pickleball, anyway? How did it become one of the fastest-growing sports in the United States, and now, the world? If you've ever pondered either (or both) of those questions, you've come to the right place! The pickleball origin story is fascinating, entertaining, and even a bit mysterious. So, let's travel back in time and learn more about the founders of this beloved game, how the first court was created, and how the sport blossomed into the phenomenon it is today.

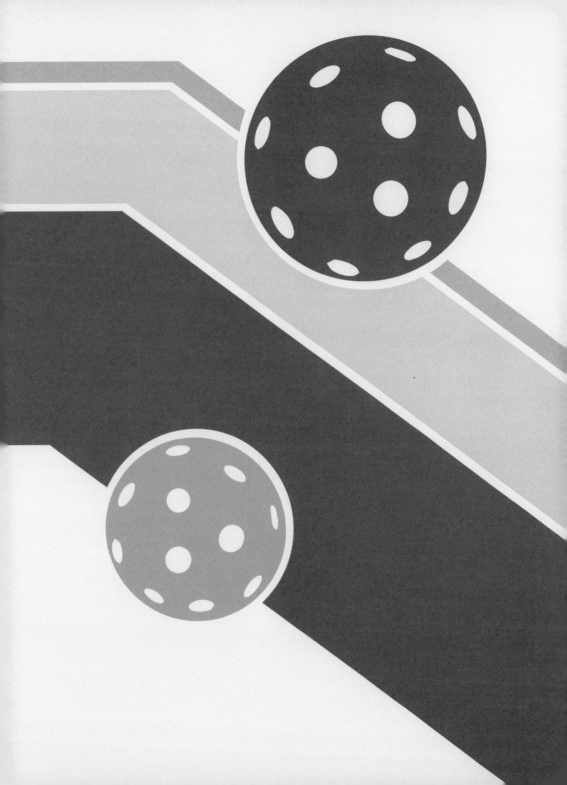

THE PICKLEBALL ORIGIN STORY

One summer afternoon in 1965, two best friends, Joel Pritchard and Bill Bell, set out with a few others to play badminton on Bainbridge Island, Washington. They found a court, but unfortunately, didn't have enough equipment for everyone to play. Instead of just cutting their losses and sulking in boredom, the two innovative friends decided to freestyle it. They grabbed some table tennis paddles and a perforated plastic ball and began volleying it over the badminton net.

While this concept seemed to work at first, they thought they could improve it by lowering the badminton net from 60 to 36 inches (0.9 to 1.5 m). If they'd left it at 60 inches, I wonder if that would have saved me from being hit in the face as many times as I have? After numerous rallies, the two friends and their families enjoyed the game so much, they introduced another friend, Barney McCallum, to the concept the following weekend.

Now, I wasn't there, but I'm sure McCallum must have raised an eyebrow when his two friends explained this new game to him. A sport that's a mixture of regular tennis, badminton, and table tennis? It definitely would have been greeted by a wide-eyed, puzzled expression from me. However, as the (now three) friends continued to play the game and share it with others, they developed some rules.

Ultimately, what was at first just a way to pass some time turned into a game the entire family could play. Pickleball continued to be played on a badminton court until 1967, when Bob O'Brien (a neighbor of Pritchard and Bell's) constructed a permanent concrete pickleball court in his own backyard. It's cool his other neighbors were okay with it too (not everyone enjoys the constant "ping" sound of a pickleball being hit with a paddle).

It took a while for pickleball to really explode—a few decades, actually—and that's okay. My dad used to tell me that college was a marathon, not a sprint, and the same applied to pickleball.

However, as word of the hybrid sport started to spread, more and more people became interested in it. Finally, in 1984, the United States Amateur Pickleball Association (USAPA) was formed to oversee the new sport, and thus, pickleball was (officially) born!

Why Is It Called Pickleball?

It's quite a funny name for a sport, pickleball. For a long time, I thought my stepdad was playing a game called "pick-up ball." If you're like me, when you first heard someone say it, you probably instantly thought of a big jar of dills. When you first heard the word "pickleball," you probably wondered how in the heck the sport ever got its name, right? It must be because Pritchard and Bell loved pickles, right? Well, while I'm sure they enjoyed consuming vinegared cucumbers as much as the next person, that doesn't appear to be how the sport got its name. As a matter of fact, no one really knows the definitive reason why or how pickleball came to be called pickleball—but there are a few theories.

One of these involves Pritchard's wife, Joan. It's said that when she noticed the similarities between the various sports that were combined to create the game, it reminded her of the common rowing term "pickle boat." A pickle boat is rowed by the oarsmen who weren't chosen to join the teams in the other boats. Picture all the kids who were always last to be picked in gym class rowing a boat and that's a pickle boat. I'm not gonna lie; I'd have ended up on the pickle boat myself, so it's a good thing I don't row.

The other theory is a bit more straightforward: Pritchard named the sport after their dog, Pickles, who enjoyed sprinting off with the ball mid-game. I like to think that Pickles was just adding a new aspect to the game and wanted some involvement in its creation. Nevertheless, "pickleball" was only implemented after the sport had gained popularity and needed an official name. At that point, it just made sense to keep it, given the unique nature of the sport.

PICKLEBALL FOR ALL

There's no question that pickleball has taken the world by storm, but how exactly did it go from being played in a Washington State backyard to one of the fastest-growing sports in the US? Well, for starters, the sport appeals to a wide demographic. Pickleball isn't for just one body type, nationality, gender, age, and so on; it's for everyone! You can even play in a wheelchair.

It's also a pretty simple game, and you don't have to be in peak physical shape to play it.

People often associate racquet sports with "elite" society. This is likely because many courts are located at

PICKLE POINTER

You can play pickleball anywhere! All you need is a portable net and some tape or chalk to create the lines.

country clubs or other exclusive facilities. Pickleball, however, is different. You can play pickleball in your driveway, the street, a parking lot, on a tennis court, or at the gym. I've even seen people catching a game at the beach! After all, all you need to play is a net, some paddles, a ball, and a few distinguishing lines.

As most nets are portable these days, the biggest obstacle is the more time-consuming effort of taping or chalking lines. Although, keeping their shoes tied while playing seems to be the bigger obstacle for some (always be sure to double-knot, folks!).

In addition to its relatively easy setup, the sport is also fairly simple to learn to play. Anyone who has decent hand-eye coordination can play pickleball. Unfortunately for my mother, this doesn't include everyone, but I'll give her credit for at least making an effort.

You can make a pickleball game as simple or as high intensity and fast paced as you'd like, but of course, this will also depend on the other players. While I consider myself to be a fairly advanced player, I still have a blast whenever I play with friends and family who are beginners.

Pickleball can be played in both singles and doubles, but most folks tend to prefer doubles due to the social aspect. Plus, if you don't enjoy constantly chasing a ball, singles matches probably aren't for you.

While the number of professional pickleball players has risen significantly in recent years, it's still mostly known as a social sport. It's perfect for those who are in the mood for a bit of socializing after a stressful day at work, or for parents who need a quick, fun activity while their children are at school.

I can't tell you how many parents I've seen roll up to the pickleball courts after dropping their kids off at school, and I don't blame them. Would you rather spend your morning cleaning up glitter-slime projects gone wrong or playing some pickleball? That choice is simple: clean up the glitter slime (kidding!).

The beauty of pickleball is you can head out to your local courts, play some music, drink some lemonade (or hard seltzer), and unwind while playing the greatest sport on Earth. Personally, I don't recommend dinking and drinking if you want to win any matches, but to each their own.

In addition to being able to play pickleball with your grandma or cousin who hasn't run a mile since high school gym class, there are many other appealing things about the sport. For example, many tennis players are transitioning to pickleball because it's less strenuous on their bodies. Instead of having to cover an entire tennis court as a lone ranger, in pickleball, you only have to cover one-fourth. Pretty convenient, right?

Also, getting hit in the face with a pickleball is a lot less painful than a tennis ball, and as I mentioned earlier, I would know—I've been hit in the face numerous times by both, and I don't even play tennis. Having a ball-magnet face isn't a pleasant experience, but you play the cards you've been dealt.

While having some sort of tennis or racquet sport experience under your belt will definitely be beneficial when

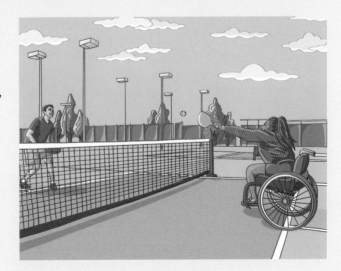

From Tennis to Pickleball via Hollywood

Professional tennis is an extremely difficult career to break into. People can start playing when they're toddlers and play all through college, but still never get the opportunity to play professionally. This is mostly due to the competitive nature of tennis, but also the level of difficulty involved in learning and improving. Many players also don't have the necessary funds to pay for the expensive coaching, tournament fees, travel expenses, hotels, and so on.

As pickleball requires a similar skill set, many high-level tennis players, including Dekel Bar, Collin Johns, Salome Devidze, and Parris Todd, have transitioned over to the sport and become some of the world's best players. (Now, if only we could get Serena Williams and Roger Federer to make the switch!)

It's not just professional tennis players who are taking up pickleball, though; pro athletes from other sports, public figures, influencers, and celebrities are also getting in on the fun. For example, Olympic swimmer Michael Phelps and former NFL players Drew Brees and Larry Fitzgerald have all started to play and promote pickleball. Brees even played a match with pickleball pro Matt Manasse against Jeb Bush while the latter's father, George W. Bush, former president of the United States, watched. That's pretty dang cool!

Hollywood has also taken an interest in pickleball. George Clooney and his wife, Amal, reportedly play on their own home court, while comedian and former talk show host Ellen DeGeneres even has her own line of pickleball paddles. An episode of *Keeping Up with the Kardashians* featured the family learning how to play the sport, and David Dobrick, influencer and creator of the Vine video platform, now competes in pickleball tournaments.

Due to the portable nature of pickleball, it's also going on tour—and I don't mean the professional pickleball tour. I'm talking about music! Country music star Dierks Bentley was actually dinking onstage with other players while belting out ballads. However, it was Brett Eldredge who took it to the next level, singing "My Girl" while simultaneously playing pickleball with some of his tour mates during a live show.

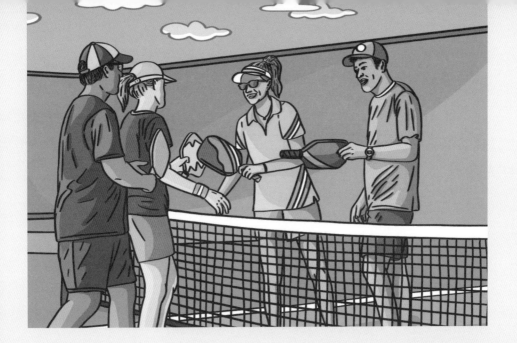

transitioning to pickleball, it isn't required. There are numerous pickleball professionals who have never played tennis.

As long as you can maneuver forward, backward, sideways, diagonally, and (in some cases) toward the sky, you have the potential to become a talented pickleball player. I can't begin to count the number of times I've had my ego tarnished on the court by someone nearly three times my age, and I played college-level lacrosse.

Pickleball is truly a sport unlike any other. It allows players to reach an advanced level, even if they're struggling with disabilities and injuries. It's strategic in nature, but also electrifying and addictive—I once sat in traffic for three hours just to play pickleball, which I never would've done for lacrosse. It also connects you with people you might not meet otherwise. Never in my wildest dreams did I imagine I would have as many good friends as I do now, and I owe it all to pickleball.

Because the sport is growing so rapidly, finding someone to practice with likely won't be an issue. The pickleball community is also extremely welcoming to new players because we were all there not that long ago and know what it's like to be the new kid on the court. I was extremely intimidated the first time

The Different Types of Pickleball Players

Pickleball has taken me to a wide range of locations throughout the world, and I have met some of the most fun, outgoing, and charming individuals on my pickleball journey. As I continue to travel, I can always count on finding these types of players at the local pickleball courts:

BANGERS

These players like to drive the ball very hard at the opposing team. There's no dinking or resetting—only huge swings at the ball from any area of the court.

SOFT GAMERS

The opposite of the bangers, these folks prefer to dink and play a "soft" game. While this might be a far less exhilarating match than you'll get with the bangers, at least you won't have to worry about losing an eye!

LOBBERS

The most annoying—but effective—players in the sport. True to their name, these are the players who lob the ball over their opponents' heads during a dinking rally, forcing you or your partner to retrieve the ball from midcourt or the baseline, and reset it (that is, hit a soft, shallow-arching shot that lands in the kitchen area).

SOCIAL PLAYERS

Arguably the most enjoyable group to hang out with, these folks usually play a few times a week but don't tend to compete in tournaments. They often show up with a cooler and a Bluetooth speaker.

HYPEBEASTS

These are the players you'll hear quoting pickleball commercials or referencing pro-player shots. Some will only play a match with a GoPro attached to their chest to capture their every move. They'll do anything to become the best player at the local court.

HOTHEADS

You'll likely hear these pickleballers before you see them. They tend to get a bit too worked up whenever anything goes awry. In tournaments, outbursts like that can earn you a fault for unsportsmanlike conduct, but during casual play, you might want to avoid them unless you enjoy being yelled at.

HECKLERS

These are the trash-talkers. During a match, they use this tactic to intimidate or discourage their opponents. It's generally best to ignore them, but gosh, wouldn't it be awful if they received a drive right to the face? Whoops!

I visited a public court. I remember putting my paddle in line at one of the challenge courts (more on this later) and playing against people who were far more advanced than I was.

After losing badly, I was worried no one would ever want to play with me again, but, to my surprise, the group took me in and taught me some new skills. Now, I play in tournaments with some of them. If they hadn't been so kind and accommodating that evening, I probably would have been too nervous to ever go back.

PICKLE POINTER

Unlike many other sports, anyone can advance to a higher level in pickleball.

If you're just starting out, this book will be your guide to the pickleball world! I'll be covering everything from recreational play and improving your game, to the different types of players you'll encounter and how to navigate your first tournament.

When I first started playing, I knew absolutely nothing about the pickleball world, but this book will give you a head start. However, do beware—you might become just as obsessed with pickleball as the rest of us!

LINGO *and* EQUIPMENT

Before you can play any sport, you have to purchase the necessary equipment. For pickleball, this includes a paddle, some pickleballs, and (most likely) a portable net. Like anything, though, there are tons of options for all of these items on the market. You'll also need to learn the lingo. In this section, I'll help you choose the right equipment and go over the terms and phrases you'll be hearing on the court.

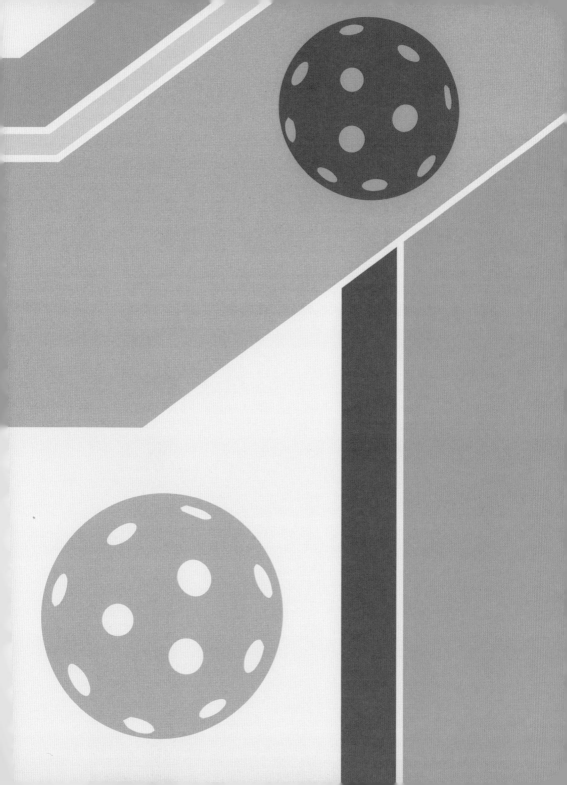

PICKLE PREP

I can sense it: Your deep desire is to just get to it and start playing pickleball already! You're just about to shout, "Put me in, Coach! I'm ready," but easy, tiger. Okay, so first, I'm not your coach, but rather, your pickleball tour guide. Also, you're probably not a tiger.

However, before you can enter the pickledome, you have to learn the basics and get suited up! If you've never played any other racquet sport before, you're going to be hearing a lot of terminology you're unfamiliar with.

When I was a newbie, pickleball lingo all sounded like gibberish to me. But instead of asking what these terms and phrases meant, I'd usually just smile and nod, pretending I knew exactly what the other person was talking about.

Again, though, this book is meant to give you a head start. After you finish this section, not only will your smile and nod when someone starts speaking pickleball be genuine, but you'll be armed with the best gear as well.

BASIC TERMINOLOGY

If you don't yet know your rallies from your runs, you might be highly confused during much of your time on the pickleball court. Like any sport, pickleball has its own lingo and terminology, and the meanings aren't always obvious. For example, when someone says (in a somber tone) "good shot" or "yeah" to their opponent after they miss a shot, it usually means they're frustrated. If someone you just played a recreational game with asks if you want to "run it back," they're asking if you want to play another.

We'll go over some of the main terms here, but I highly recommend you visit the Glossary before moving forward so you won't be lost in later sections. Familiarizing yourself with the language of pickleball will not only give you a better understanding of the game, but it'll also "erne" you (wink) some major points with your fellow players.

Of course, you *could* just throw around some of the terms you've heard without really knowing what they mean. However, you'll likely get some strange looks from players in the know, followed by some awkward conversations.

Relax—you're not going to be tested on this. There's no need to make flash cards or worry about a pop quiz.

Simply peruse the Glossary and the definitions below, and you'll soon speak fluent pickletalk:

DINK RESPONSIBLY

- **Dink:** When you hit the ball as lightly as possible at (or near) the net, so it's just high enough to go over, but low enough that your opponent(s) can't hit it from the air.
- **Ground stroke:** The most common stroke in all of pickleball, this is simply hitting the ball after it bounces.
- **Hands battle:** A series of fast volleys back and forth from the kitchen line between two players or teams.
- **The kitchen or non-volley zone (NVZ):** The area of the court that is 7 feet (2.1 m) from both sides of the net, and from sideline to sideline.
- **Lob:** The most dreaded shot in all of pickleball, this is when you hit the ball so high into the air, it sails right over your opponent(s). An effective lob soars to the back of the court, forcing one (or both) of the players to chase it backward to retrieve it.
- **Rally:** A point that's played out from the moment the ball is served until there's a fault.
- **Run:** A series of points won consecutively by the serving team.
- **Volley:** When a ball is hit in the air before it hits the ground during a rally.

Great job, dinker! You're now on your way to becoming a pickleball encyclopedia. Even if you never play pickleball again and just watch matches on TV, you'll know exactly what the commentators are talking about. And yes, I heard that gasp. *Never play pickleball again?!* Of course you will.

First, though, it's time to jump online and buy yourself a snazzy new pickleball paddle!

CHOOSING THE RIGHT PADDLE

Some players say "it's the player, not the paddle," but I believe selecting the perfect paddle can have a major influence on how you play. For example, if your paddle is too heavy for you, you might struggle when returning to your "ready position" for the next shot. Additionally, if you hit your strokes with backspin, then a carbon-fiber surface could really elevate your game.

When you first start shopping for a paddle, though, you may quickly be overwhelmed with the vast number of choices and options. They come in so many different grits, lengths, and weights, you might wonder if you need to worry about *all* of those things. You'll also see more than a few that claim to be "the most powerful paddle on the market," but they can't all be, can they? And why are some of them so expensive?

Choosing the right pickleball paddle is similar to choosing the right wand before you head to Hogwarts. However, when you've found just the right one, you'll wonder how you ever made it this far without it.

The key to finding the right paddle is to test them out. If you live in an area that actually has a brick-and-mortar pickleball store, go there instead of shopping online. They usually have "demo" paddles you can try out before purchasing. Many online pickleball shops will also allow you a trial period with a paddle before you make your final purchase. Another option is to head to your local courts. Someone will most likely let you hit a few balls with their paddle if you tell them you're on the hunt for a new one.

You know those people who always need to have the latest, greatest version of whatever they're into (iPhones, cars, laptops, and so on)? Well, pickleball is no different. There's always likely to be at least one paddle collector at your local courts, and they always have the newest, most cutting-edge model. But that's good news for you! Due to their continuous quest for the new, these players are often selling very lightly used paddles at a discount.

Once you find one you like, you can either find a local ambassador for that brand who might have a discount code or order online from a major paddle retailer. If you're interested in finding a local ambassador, try reaching out to the paddle company's customer service via phone or social media; they should be able to provide you with a list of ambassadors in your area.

Will You Be Using Your Paddle in Tournaments?

If you plan to take your pickleball game all the way to the tournament circuit, certain leagues require you to have a paddle that's USA Pickleball approved. Any model that is will have a stamp above the handle that says "USAPA approved" or "USA Pickleball approved."

This means that the paddle was submitted to USA Pickleball by the paddle manufacturer, tested, inspected, and approved for tournament usage. To qualify, the paddle's surface area (including the length, width, and edge guard) must not exceed 24 inches (61 cm). Its length also cannot exceed 17 inches (43 cm), and the width should complement the length.

Other factors that are reviewed include the material(s) the paddle is made of, its surface roughness, and mechanical features. For the full list of requirements a paddle must meet to be USA Pickleball–approved, visit the USA Pickleball website (usapickleball.org).

If you just plan to use your paddle strictly for recreational play, you can snag any design your little heart desires. Some of the more aesthetic models come in the cutest designs.

One of the advantages of buying a paddle directly from the brand's website is that it can be easier for the company to look up your information, track your order, and replace it if the equipment breaks due to a manufacturing error. If you're a hothead who tends to chuck your paddle ten yards every time you miss a put-away (i.e., a shot that's intentionally very difficult for the opposition to hit), then, most likely, your paddle will not be replaced every time you break it. Handle your equipment with care and dink responsibly. With paddle price tags ranging from $25 to nearly $350, it's important that you make the right selection.

But keep in mind (and I'm speaking from experience here), just because a paddle is expensive doesn't mean you're going to play any better. So let's cover the most important things you should consider.

PADDLE MATERIALS

Paddles can be made of four materials: wood, composite, graphite, or carbon fiber. Wood is the cheapest option, but they're also the least used, because they're heavy and tend to break easily. Also, splinters are no fun! I would never play a serious pickleball game with a wooden paddle—leave them for the middle school gym classes.

Composite paddles are the middle-of-the-road option. Made primarily of fiberglass, their texture can be ideal for generating spin and power. Also, because fiberglass isn't nearly as stiff as some of the other materials, composite paddles are like boomerangs. They absorb the energy from the ball, and then use it to bounce the ball off the paddle. Crikey! The weight of composite paddles is midrange, making them ideal for all types of players.

Most high-quality and luxury paddles are made of graphite due to its lighter weight and durability. These paddles can also add more power and control to your game, and their lighter weight makes them ideal for players who are prone to tennis elbow. If you tend to plop up your dinks, or often try to hit the ball one way and it goes another, then a graphite paddle is for you. The only downside is they tend to be a bit pricier than the wood or composite options, but totally worth the investment, in my opinion.

Carbon-fiber paddles are a bit newer to pickleball, but they're known for their ability to generate spin due to their rough surface and maximum power. Due to these attributes, they are every pickleball banger's weapon of choice. Recently, nearly every paddle manufacturer has released a carbon-fiber model. The material is very stiff, so the energy of the ball is spread throughout the entire paddle rather than confined to just a small area.

PADDLE WEIGHT AND THICKNESS

Most pickleball paddles weigh anywhere from 4 to 14 ounces (113 to 397 g). The heavier the paddle (anything over 10 ounces, or 283 g), the more power it generates. Seasoned tennis players are ideal candidates for heavier paddles. A lighter paddle (anything from 6 to 8 ounces, or 170 to 227 g), on the other hand, offers more control and is easier to swing. If you've had any arm injuries or are prone to tennis elbow, I don't recommend playing with a heavier paddle, as this could cause you more pain and/or irritate your injury. A midweight paddle (7 to 9 ounces, or 198 to 255 g) is ideal for those who are looking for a balance of power and control.

Some players add lead tape to their paddles around the edge guard to make them heavier. Depending on where you add it, though, it can affect how the paddle plays. I add lead tape to the bottom half of my paddle, near the handle, for additional stability. If you choose a paddle with a lot of power, just keep in mind you might be sacrificing control, and a lot of your pickleballs might end up soaring clear to the parking lot.

When selecting a paddle, you'll also typically notice a measurement in millimeters (mm) listed. This refers to the core thickness of the paddle; the thicker the core, the more stable it will be. A thin core would be anything from 10 to 14 millimeters, while 16 millimeters or higher falls into the thicker category. A thicker core softens the feeling of the ball as it comes off your paddle and allows you more control, which helps tremendously when resetting the ball. Many defensive players prefer thicker paddles.

However, if you crave more power and pop, a thinner core would be ideal, as it allows the ball to bounce off the paddle more quickly. A paddle with a thinner core is better for offensive players, but if you have a tendency to mishit, I wouldn't recommend a thinner core.

HANDLE LENGTH AND GRIP

The current USA Pickleball rules require paddles to not exceed 17 inches (43 cm) in length, but the ratio from handle length to paddle face does not matter. Due to this, you will find that some paddles have longer handles than others. A paddle with a longer handle can generate a lot more power and spin. Many tennis players gravitate toward them, as they feel more like a tennis racquet. Plus, if (like me) you have a two-handed backhand, a longer handle will be beneficial.

Shorter handles provide more control, so many beginners and intermediate players use them. Table-tennis players also tend to use shorter handles, as they can "choke up" on the head of the paddle, with one finger behind the head, like pro pickleball player Callan Dawson.

The grip on a paddle might seem like a minor consideration, but it's just as important as any other factor. If the grip size is too large, it can cause the paddle to slip during gameplay and lead to elbow injury. Larger grip sizes are ideal for more stability, while smaller sizes offer more control. With the latter, you also have more ability to spin the ball with your wrist action. When in doubt, I recommend going for a smaller grip size. You can always add layers of overgrip to increase the size if you need to.

Overgrip is a soft, cloth-like tape you can wrap around the grip of your paddle to provide extra cushioning. This will not only reduce blisters, but it also provides tackiness and sweat absorption. I typically change out the overgrip on my paddle at least once a week, depending on how often I'm playing and the climate in which I'll be playing. This is necessary because, over time, overgrip loses its tackiness and will no longer absorb sweat.

When your paddle starts slipping and sliding in your hand, it's time to change your overgrip. If you use a lighter-colored overgrip, you'll also notice a color change. In fact, it might turn black from sweat and dirt (yuck!). This is a great reminder to wash and sanitize your hands after practice. Those pickleballs can pick up a lot of dirt.

An elongated paddle is generally anything over 16 inches (40 cm) long and around 7 inches (17.5 cm) wide. The Electrum Model E, Joola Hyperion, and Selkirk Vanguard are all good examples of elongated paddles. Maneuverability can be more difficult with an elongated paddle, but you'll have much more reach and power. This makes them the most beneficial paddles for players who regularly take balls out of the air behind the kitchen at the non-volley zone, and those who play singles.

However, their sweet spot is also smaller—this is the area on a paddle (usually, the center) from which a player gets the most accurate contact with the ball, so it might take a few practices to adjust to these models.

A wider paddle is typically around 8½ inches (22 cm) wide with a length of 15½ inches (39 cm). They have the largest sweet spots, making them more forgiving of mishits and ideal for newer players. They're also much whippier than elongated paddles, so it's easier to generate power and control. The Electrum Pro and CRBN^2 are good examples of wide paddles.

TEXTURE AND SHAPE

Like pickleball players, paddles come in different shapes and sizes. A paddle's shape can help with power and maneuverability. A paddle's texture is also important, as it is one of the key factors for generating spin on a pickleball. For this reason, paddle manufacturers have recently started using carbon fiber on the surfaces. Spinning is important because it can limit your opponent's shot selection. It can also cause the ball to curve in the air, skid when it hits the ground (whee!), or even jump in an odd direction.

While spin can be generated by paddles with a smooth texture, one with some grit can give you a real advantage in your game. Because of this, however, there's a limit to the amount of grit a pickleball paddle can have. If you purchase a USA Pickleball–approved paddle, this will ensure it generates just enough spin to still be considered illegal. Well, in theory, that is.

In April 2022, there was a pickleball scandal involving this very thing! A paddle that was previously USA Pickleball approved tested over the grit limit. As a result, all of the brand's paddles were removed from the USAPA-approved list during one of the largest tournaments of the year because the amount of grit on the paddles was enough to significantly alter the way the ball moved, due to the spin generated. They've since been adjusted and reapproved; however, the Professional Pickleball Association (PPA) tour has now implemented paddle testing for professional players.

If a player believes their opponent's paddle is illegal, they can challenge it and have it tested on-site at the referee desk. If the paddle is found to be illegal, that player forfeits the match. It's also not a great look for the player *or* the paddle manufacturer.

HOW OFTEN SHOULD YOU REPLACE YOUR PADDLE?

Depending on how frequently you play pickleball, you might, at some point, have to replace your paddle. I know, I know; it can be hard to let your paddle go! You've won a lot of games together, so it's perfectly understandable that you've become emotionally attached. If you're a recreational player and only play a few games each week, a durable paddle can last you anywhere from two to three years. Some pro players, however, switch out their paddle every few tournaments to ensure they always have an optimal one for gameplay. And if you're extra, like some pickleball pros, you might even switch out your paddle every day of a tournament.

The more games you play with a paddle, the less durable it becomes. Most of the time, you'll know when you need a new one, though. The edge guard will likely become loose, or the once-rough surface will be smooth. Or you might hear an odd thump when you hit the ball or notice that striking it just doesn't feel the same as it did when your paddle was new. While breaking up with a pickleball paddle can be hard to do, your game will thank you.

> ### PICKLE POINTER
>
> If the edge guard on your paddle has come loose, or it just doesn't feel as comfortable as it once did when you hit the ball, it's time to shop for a new one.

PICKLEBALLS

Pickleballs are all the same, right? Wrong. While, yes, they're all essentially plastic Wiffle balls, there are several differences. Like your paddle, one thing you'll want to consider when selecting a pickleball is whether it's USA Pickleball approved. Again, this will ensure that you're prepared if you ever want to play in a league or tournament.

To be USA Pickleball approved, a ball has
to meet the following specifications:

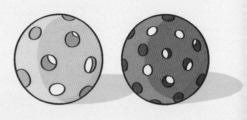

- Made of plastic
- Weigh between 0.78 and 0.935 ounces
  (22.1 and 26.5 g)
- Measure 2.874 to 2.972 inches (7.3
  to 7.5 cm) in diameter

If you're ever training for a tournament, you'll definitely want to make sure
you're playing with the same ball you'll be using when you compete. The
tournament's website will always specify the type of pickleball that will be used.

There are also two main types of pickleballs: indoor and outdoor. Indoor
pickleballs are meant for playing on gym flooring or clay courts. They're more
textured and much thicker than outdoor balls to help you generate spin. The
holes are also larger than those on outdoor balls, and there are fewer of them.

Because they move slower than the outdoor variety, smashing an indoor ball
for a good put-away can be difficult. However, they're extremely durable; I don't
think I've ever seen anyone break an indoor pickleball by hitting it too hard.
Maybe pickleball pro Daniel de la Rosa will attempt this at some point. He has
the most powerful overhead smash I've ever seen—and it's terrifying. Of course,
he's one of the world's top-ranked racquetball players, so it makes sense.

Due to their lighter weight, indoor balls aren't ideal for outdoor use. They're
just too impacted by wind. So, next time your friend whips out an indoor ball
for an outdoor game, politely suggest that you use an outdoor ball. Or you can
cringe and give them a look of complete disgust—up to you!

Because I live in a warmer climate, I don't play too often indoors or on
clay-surface courts. However, if you do, I'd recommend the DuraFast, Onix Fuse,
or Gamma Photon indoor pickleballs. They're all USA Pickleball approved for
sanctioned tournament play.

Outdoor pickleballs have more holes than indoor pickleballs, and these
holes are smaller; whereas indoor pickleballs have twenty-six or so holes, the
outdoor kind have forty, which allow the ball to move faster through the air and
not be as affected by wind. Although outdoor pickleballs are heavier, they wear
out much faster than indoor balls. The more you play with one, the easier it will

be to break. The plastic also expands in hotter temperatures, making the ball "mushy" and harder to put away. In colder temperatures, it will harden and break more easily. If you play in cooler temperatures, I recommend the Franklin X-40 because a DuraFast 40 will break too easily (and pickleballs can be pricey).

Another thing that can decrease the lifespan of a pickleball is the

PICKLE POINTER

Just because you're playing indoors doesn't mean you have to use indoor pickleballs. Many indoor facilities now have typical outdoor surfaces on their courts, so you can use outdoor pickleballs.

surface on which you play; asphalt or concrete might cause the ball to lose its shape and become lopsided pretty fast. If you notice your pickleball is moving oddly, check to make sure it's still spherical and hasn't become lopsided.

The outdoor pickleballs I use during practice are the Onix DuraFast 40 and Franklin Sports X-40. Both of these are used in the tournaments in which I compete, so I find it extremely beneficial to use them when preparing for competition. If you also plan to compete, I recommend you pick up a few of each of these.

Although yellow and neon green are the most common for visibility—especially in professional or sanctioned tournaments—pickleballs come in nearly every color imaginable. Some people even use the more colorful options as home décor.

Instead of trashing them, some folks repurpose their old pickleballs as Christmas ornaments or wreath accents. (I once saw a Christmas tree made entirely out of pickleballs!) You can also paint cracked pickleballs and turn them into centerpieces for various holidays, or even attach one to your car antenna!

Unfortunately, when thrown in the trash, they just end up in landfills. If arts and crafts aren't your thing, you can also recycle your pickleballs. I've probably cracked nearly one hundred pickleballs at this point, and I used to just throw them away like everyone else. Now I have a bin in my garage that is my ball graveyard. Whenever it's full, I empty the dead balls in a bag and take them to the local recycling center.

PORTABLE NETS

Not everyone is fortunate enough to have permanent pickleball courts down at the local sports park. Also, as tennis players don't want their courts permanently converted for pickleball (and some are annoyed by the "pinging" sounds of the sport), many cities are reluctant to do so. The compromise that's been reached in some locations has been to add pickleball lines to public tennis courts and to only allow play during certain hours of the day. In fact, the lines for two pickleball courts can be added to every one tennis court without disrupting anyone's game. Plus, when tennis players see all the fun the pickleball players are having, they'll want to join in!

Even if your local tennis court has pickleball lines, you're going to need a portable, temporary net to practice. Luckily, they're definitely not a hassle to put together at all. Why, you'll *never* find yourself screaming in frustration after you realize you put the holes together backward and now have to tear the whole thing down and start over. Okay, so maybe my sarcasm was a bit overly dramatic there.

Assembling portable nets isn't *that* bad. Some even come with the poles tethered together, so you don't have to guess which one connects to which. It only takes about five to ten minutes to assemble one, but you'll be having hours of fun afterward! Until, of course, you have to disassemble the net.

One major benefit of using a portable net is its more flexible design—even if the ball hits the top of the net, it will likely still land on the opposite side. These shots are sure to frustrate your opponents because they're hard to react to; they either barely trickle over the net or they continue flying, but in an unpredictable path. As a result, it's common courtesy to raise a hand and apologize whenever this happens, unless it's the match point; then, by all means, go ahead and shake your tail feathers!

✳✳✳

So, now that you've learned the lingo and bought the necessary equipment, it's time to play pickleball, right? Well . . . you should probably learn the rules first.

GAME BASICS

In this section, you'll get a very basic overview of how to play pickleball. However, just like any sport, keep in mind that there are many aspects you can explore far beyond the basic rules of the game. The intent of this section is just to get you going, and it's a stellar starting point for anyone who is just beginning their pickleball journey.

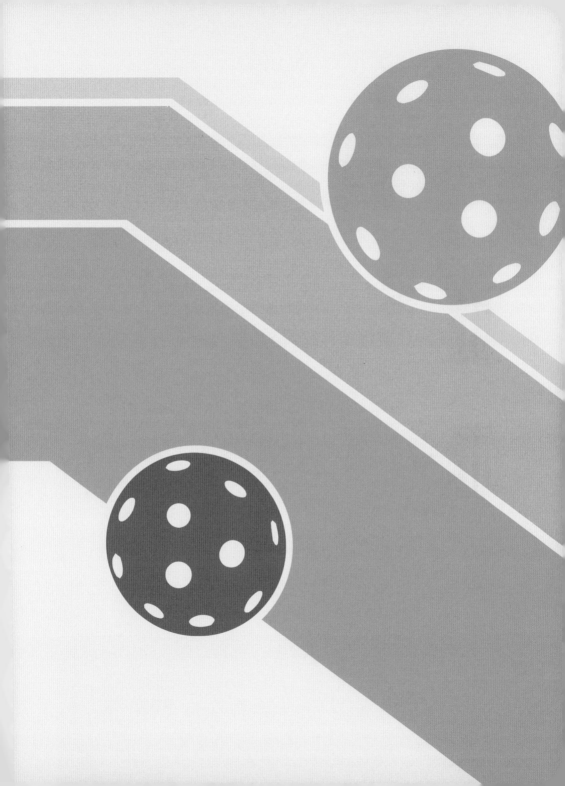

YOU HAVE TO LEARN BEFORE YOU CAN LOB

"Excuse me, lady, but we came here to learn pickleball!" Sheesh, I get it! You're an eager student, and I'm also quite flattered that you came to me to learn about pickleball. I almost feel like a pickleball Yoda, except I'm not nearly as wise, intuitive, or good looking.

Still, I'm glad I Jedi mind-tricked you into playing the greatest sport of all time. Okay, maybe I'm overreaching a bit there, but I think you've made a wise decision. Now, we're going to take a deep dive into what the pickleball court looks like, some of the basic rules, how scoring works, and how the heck you actually play this game.

May the lob be with you, young overhead smasher.

THE COURT

The first thing you need to play pickleball is a court. If there aren't any permanent options near you, no worries—most of the top pickleball professionals started out playing with portable nets on temporary courts.

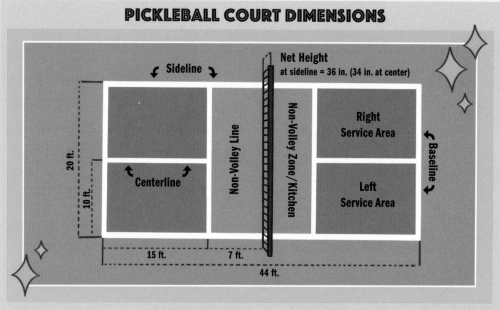

PICKLEBALL COURT DIMENSIONS

Sideline

Net Height
at sideline = 36 in. (34 in. at center)

Non-Volley Line

Non-Volley Zone / Kitchen

Right
Service Area

Baseline

20 ft.

Centerline

Left
Service Area

10 ft.

15 ft.   7 ft.

44 ft.

Play Area: 30 x 60 ft. (min. recommended)

Pickleball is played on a rectangular-shaped court that measures 44 feet (13 m) long by 20 feet (6 m) wide. The net is placed in the center, and on either side there's a line 7 feet (2.1 m) from the net called the "non-volley zone" or, more commonly, "the kitchen." Now, you're probably wondering why on earth it's called that. Maybe because the kitchen is where the pickles are?

Well, once again, I'll have to give you a theory about that because there's no precise answer. Some people think the term was borrowed from shuffleboard, in which the kitchen is the area before the scoring zone, but no one knows for sure.

The surface of the court is the same as an outdoor tennis or basketball court and textured with a nonaggressive silica sand to provide a nonslip, smooth surface. While this texture is supposed to prevent you from slipping in wet conditions, I wouldn't recommend playing pickleball when the courts are wet. You could seriously injure yourself.

Some indoor pickleball facilities have started placing a rubbery polyurethane (big word alert) mat over their flat, concrete flooring. This can be advantageous for indoor play, as it provides some cushioning for players and helps reduce stress on knees and joints.

Other indoor pickleball courts have polished, wooden gym floors (think middle school gym class). These types of courts are predominantly found at community sports centers. Typically, pickleball court lines are painted on the basketball court, but you'll usually have to to use a portable net. Many indoor pickleball tournaments are geared toward players who prefer a gym floor to an outdoor surface. As pickleball continues to grow in popularity, more clay, and even grass courts, have started popping up as well.

You might have started to see pickleball courts in various bright colors, which is a glorious thing! Pickleball courts aren't restricted to any certain color, but blue is quite common for courts because of the contrast it offers for yellow and green pickleballs. Beige and green is another popular combination because it blends in with the landscape.

Now that you're familiar with the glorious pickleball court (isn't she beautiful?), it's time to dig into those rules.

THE RULES OF PICKLEBALL

Once you've arrived at the pickleball court and properly stretched and hydrated, it's time to get playing! Like any game or sport, learning how to play pickleball can be a bit overwhelming at first, but once you play a few times, you'll catch on fairly easily. One thing to keep in mind with pickleball is that, because it's a relatively new sport, the rules are still evolving. This is especially true at the competitive level, but you can always check the Rulebook section at usapickleball.org for any updates.

In this section, we'll go over scoring, serving, the return, the infamous third shot, and what it means to "play out a point."

FORMAT AND SCORING

Pickleball can be played in either a singles (two players) or doubles (four players) format. Mixed doubles is when there's a man and a woman on both teams. The rules of the game are the same for both doubles and singles, but as I mentioned previously, chasing that plastic Wiffle ball around a court in a singles game doesn't appeal to most folks. As doubles is the more popular way to play, I'll explain the rules as they would apply for four players. Keep in mind, though, you'll score some major brownie points (and respect) from your peers if you play singles. You'll also have an excuse to treat yourself to a double scoop of ice cream after practice (just sayin').

Scoring in pickleball can be slightly confusing at first, but the overall objective is pretty simple: the first team to get 11 points wins; however, you have to win by 2 points. For example, if the score is 10–10 and you score another point for 11, you still need to get

> ### PICKLE POINTER
> Before a serve, three numbers must always be called: the server's score, the receiver's score, and the number of the player serving the ball.

one more for a total of 12 to win. You can also only score points when your team is serving. To score points while you're serving, the receiving team has to hit a ball out of bounds, make a fault, hit the ball into their side of the net, or miss the serving shot completely.

So, whenever you're trying a new shot or play, the best time to do so is when your team is serving. Then, if you make an error, at least you won't lose any points. Unfortunately, if you miss your serve, either hitting the ball out of bounds or into the net, you don't get to play out the point and the ball goes to the next server.

Before serving the ball, three numbers are called by the server or referee (if one is present): the server's score, the receiver's score, and (if playing doubles) the server's number. For example, if the score is 10–9–2, the team serving has 10 points, the team receiving has 9 points, and the player serving the ball is the second server. For a score of 7–3–1, the serving team has 7 points, the receiving team has 3 points, and the player serving the ball is the first server.

The first server continues to serve until the point is lost, and then the second server takes over. This often elicits some groans from the other side of the net if the serving team just went on a "run," meaning they just scored several points in a row. Once that

The Advantage of Stacking

Recently, "stacking" has become a common practice in pickleball games. This means, instead of playing "straight-up" (switching positions throughout the game depending on the score), you rearrange your team to keep a player on one side of the court. Some folks play better on the left and some play better on the right. While most are comfortable on both sides, there's usually one side of the court on which a player is more consistent.

If you're an aggressive player, the left side will likely be best for you because it will allow you to take more forehand shots in the middle. If you prefer defense and resetting, the right side of the court might be ideal, so you can set up your partner for the attacks.

A team that has both a left- and a right-handed player would want to stack so both of their forehands are in the middle. This means the leftie would be on the right side of the court and the right-handed player would be on the left. Stacking is also a great way to disguise your weaknesses and maximize your strengths. Just remember, if you choose to stack, always make sure you're in the correct position to avoid a fault.

point is lost, though, it's "side-out" (i.e., the serving team loses the ball), and the first server on the other team gets to take their turn. For singles scoring, only the server and receiver scores are called.

Also, an easy way to keep track of the score is by referencing your player position. Let's say it's a new a new game and you're playing straight-up (so, not stacking). The score is 0–0–2 and player 1 is the starting server on the right side, while their partner, player 2, is starting on the left. Player 1 serves the ball and your team ends up winning the rally. Player 1 would then move to the left service box, player 2 would move to the right, and the score is now odd, 1–0–2.

Again, you win the rally after player 1 serves, and both players move back to their starting positions. The score now is 2–0–2. As you can see, if player 1 is standing on the right side, then the score must be even. If player 1 is standing on the left side, then the score must be odd.

SERVING

If you're serving the ball, you must call the score before the ball makes contact with your paddle, or you will receive a fault. If a game has a referee, they will call the score. If the incorrect score is called by the server or referee, any player can stop the point prior to a return being hit. If the incorrect score was called, the correct score should be called, and then there will be a re-serve, but no penalty. If the correct score was called, however,

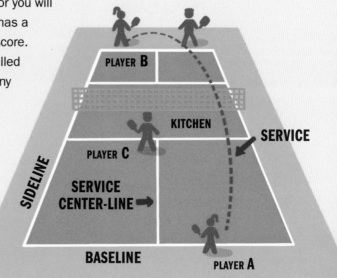

then the player who stopped the game receives a fault and the rally is lost.

This rule tends to apply more in a tournament setting, but it's still important to know. I can't tell you how many times I've been on a court with three other highly educated adults and not a single one of us can remember the score or who's serving. During recreational play, it's common courtesy to simply correct the server after the point is played out.

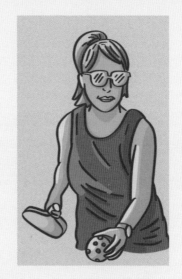

To start a game, the server must stand with both feet behind the baseline of the court prior to making contact with the ball. Countless players (myself included) have received a fault simply for having one toe on the baseline while serving. And I'm not gonna lie; this will definitely bruise your ego during a tournament match. (You'll probably also get a frustrated eye roll from your partner.)

The ball must also be served underhand (i.e., hit from below by the paddle and below the server's waistline) and hit diagonally across the court to the receiving team. The ball *must* land within the opposite diagonal service box and not touch the kitchen line. The ball can touch the center-, side-, or baselines and still be considered in.

However, you'll often hear players call the following terms during a game, all of which are out:

- **Short:** A serve that lands in the kitchen or touches the kitchen line.
- **Wide:** A serve that lands in the wrong service box or outside the sideline.
- **Back:** A ball that lands outside the baseline.

Unlike tennis, you only get one attempt at serving, but again, in a doubles game, both you and your partner will get a chance to serve before it's side-out.

It might be frustrating at first for many folks to learn how to serve underhand. The motion can feel a bit odd. Even if you've played tennis, it likely won't help much, as most players serve by throwing the ball over their head first to give it as much power as possible when they hit it.

If you find yourself struggling with the odd motion of hitting an underhand serve with your paddle in one hand and the ball in the other, you're certainly not alone. It took me nearly a month to get my serve into the correct square (yes, an *entire* month). Now, though, serving is not only one of my greatest strengths, but it's also what I'm proudest of as a player. Ace, ace, baby!

Luckily, though, there's now another serving option. The USA Pickleball Association recently started permitting drop serves. To perform a drop serve, you just drop the ball directly in front of you, and then hit it when it bounces off the ground. However, the ball must make contact with your paddle below your waistline, right around your belly button. If you don't have a belly button, feel free to serve however you like because you must be an extraterrestrial, in which case, our strange human rules do not apply.

In a tournament, the serving team is determined via a coin toss. In recreational play, though, some pickleball clubs will have unofficial rules to determine which side serves first. As of this writing, according to the USA Pickleball Association, if you serve a ball and it hits the net and then lands in the diagonal square (also known as a "let"), this doesn't result in a serve redo, and the point is played out from there. However, you always want to sure to review a tournament's rules prior to competing in case there have been any updates or changes.

THE RETURN

After a ball is served, the receiving team *must* let it bounce just once before hitting a return. The same rule applies when the ball is returned to the serving team—it must bounce once before they can hit it. The only exception to this rule is in an adaptive or wheelchair pickleball game, in which the ball is allowed to bounce twice on that side of the net.

The only other time a ball is required to bounce before you can hit it is when it's hit from inside the kitchen. This prevents players from just standing at the net and volleying every ball that comes at them.

After the first two shots have been taken and the ball has bounced, it's in free play, and you can volley from anywhere on the court behind the kitchen line. I don't recommend volleying from the baseline at any time; if a ball makes it that far, it's probably heading to the back fence and giving you an opportunity to win the point! I know it's tempting to smash that ball, but it's a lot easier to just duck out of the way. Then, you won't risk losing the point by mishitting the ball or dragging out the point any longer than necessary.

THE THIRD SHOT

After the serve and return has been hit, the serving team is responsible for the third shot. There are three common types of third shots: a drive, drop, or lob. Tennis and other racquet sport enthusiasts tend to gravitate toward the third-shot drive. This is because it has a lot of power and can win the rally against newer players who haven't yet developed strong blocking skills. If you notice one of the players on the opposing team doesn't handle pace or power

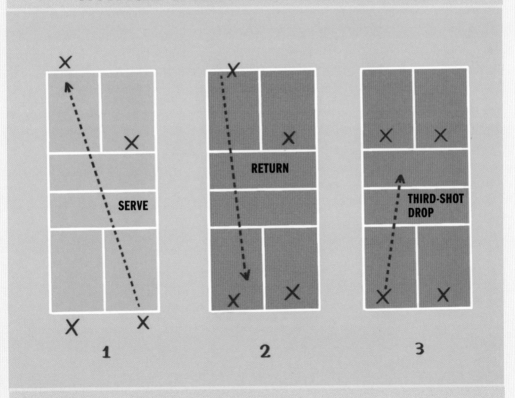

A TYPICAL OPENING PICKLEBALL SEQUENCE

SERVE

RETURN

THIRD-SHOT DROP

1

2

3

very well, or hits the ball high up after receiving a drive, this makes for an easy put-away shot afterward. A third-shot drive would be the optimal shot to take.

The third-shot drop, on the other hand, is (arguably) one of the most difficult shots in all of pickleball, given the pace and spin on the ball upon return. You'll even see many professionals miss this shot under pressure because any high drop could potentially be costly. A third-shot drop is really just a drop shot. You hit the ball in a way that gives it an arch with the goal of dropping it somewhere within the non-volley zone (the kitchen). Hitting the perfect, unattackable third-shot drop can be quite the challenge. You'll know you hit a bad one when the ball comes slamming back at your feet from one of your opponents at the kitchen line.

I once asked pickleball pro Jessie Irvine for her advice on making a third shot. She recommended that you always aim for your opponent's shoulders. This will ensure that the ball drops from its highest point at a pace that is difficult to attack. Practice this move for a while, and then definitely give it a go in-game because it absolutely works!

Another helpful tip to make a successful third-shot drop is to bend your knees to get under the ball, and then "lift" it to the appropriate height. This will also prevent you from sending your pickleball to the International Space Station. You want to shift your weight forward to the balls of your feet, and then imagine you're guiding the ball where you want it to go. I always advise players to try to be as fluid as possible.

THE THIRD-SHOT LOB

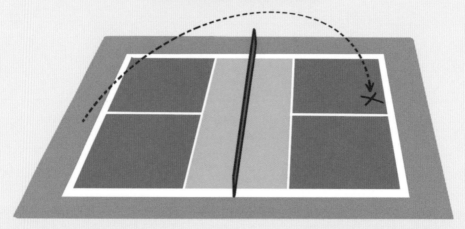

As you hold your paddle dropped with a slightly closed face (i.e., the front slightly tilted downward), keep your head down and track the pickleball as it makes contact. After I hit my third shot, a slight hop is all it takes to get me back to "ready" position—an open, forward stance with both feet facing the net. I also say a little prayer that the ball lands at a reasonable height that won't destroy my partner and me.

A third-shot lob is a lob made after the return, and you can thank pickleball pro AJ Koller for its meteoric rise in popularity. Almost all players are taught to rush the kitchen line after returning the ball to meet your partner, who will already be there. As your opponents wait at the kitchen line for either a drive or a drop, the third-shot lob can be a highly effective way to get them out of position.

If you're a beginner or intermediate player, direct your third shots toward the middle of the court, as this allows for more margin of error. I know it looks so cool when advanced players drive balls down the line or hit aggressive third-shot drops to the corner of the kitchen, but I'd rather you get the point! As you continue to play and gain more control over the ball, you can start experimenting with different placement on the court.

PLAYING OUT THE POINT

The fourth and sixth shots hit by the receiving team will most likely be aggressive to keep you and your partner back and to keep them at an advantageous position on the court. This means resetting (any shot that drops the ball in the kitchen) will be your best response.

If your third-shot drop wasn't perfect and was still attackable, it's time to use the fifth or even seventh shots to get you and your partner up to the kitchen line. Practicing drops from midcourt can help with this. Note that driving the ball from midcourt isn't always the best idea, as you're playing with a shorter distance to the baseline, so your ball is much more likely to go out of bounds.

Once both teams have reached the kitchen line, this is where the remainder of the rally will mostly be played out. It continues until someone hits a forced error (a shot that causes the other team to mess up), an unforced error (someone just messes up), or a clean winner (no one on the opposing side hits the ball).

STROKES AND SHOTS

In pickleball, there are a series of shots and strokes you can make throughout a rally. Selecting the right one at the right moment can be the difference between winning or losing the point. As you improve, so will your shot selections. Primarily, the three strokes you'll use in pickleball (which you'll also recognize from the earlier section on vocab) are the ground stroke, dink, and volley.

The ground stroke is by far the most common in pickleball and it's simply hitting the ball after it bounces. A dink, once again, is essentially a ground stroke hit near (or at) the net, but as lightly as possible.

A volley is when you hit the ball in midair before it has a chance to bounce. My favorite volley to hit is a forehand roll because it generates a lot of topspin and can be difficult for many players to return if they don't get under the ball enough. It's probably obvious from the name, but you *do not* hit a volley in the non-volley zone. Typically, volleys are more powerful shots because there's no bounce to absorb any of the ball's pace. A series of fast-paced volleys between opponents at the kitchen line is referred to as a hands battle.

Below are some of shots you'll hear about (and see) the most in pickleball:

- **Lob:** The most dreaded shot in all of pickleball, this is when the ball is hit high up into the air and sails right over the heads of your opponents. An effective lob soars to the back of the court, forcing one of the players to chase it backward to retrieve it. Lobs are mostly used as offensive shots to get the opposing team away from the kitchen line, so you can hold it (more on this later).
- **Overhead smash:** This is a volley that's hit from directly above your head. They're very difficult shots to retrieve. To

hit an overhead smash, align your body with the ball with one foot facing forward. When the ball makes contact with your paddle, swing downward. Smash!

- **Crosscourt dink:** The most common type of dink, this is when you hit a dink from one corner, across the middle of the net, to the other corner of the court. Due to the greater distance the ball has to travel, you have a 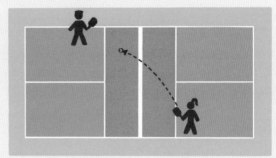 longer reaction time. The ball is also going over the lowest part of the net (the middle), so it's less likely to hit it than a down-the-line dink.
- **Counterattack:** This is an aggressive return volley shot after an opponent sends the same your way. If you're the one who attacks first, just know the ball is going to come back at you even harder and faster. The most effective counterattack is one you're able to hit at your opponent's feet rather than head-on.
- **Drive:** This is when you return either a ground stroke or a volley to your opponent as hard as you can. Tennis players love this shot, as they typically have the mechanics to hit it effectively. The most efficient time to hit a drive is when you see a court opening, or your opponent is off-balance or still running.
- **Blocking:** This is a volley used to take the pace off a drive. An effective block will reset the ball to a point low enough on the court that if your opponent tries to drive it again, it will sail out of bounds.
- **Down-the-line dink:** This is a dink you hit directly to the person in front of you, and it tends to make your opponent(s) the most uncomfortable. It gives them a shorter reaction time, in addition to the fact that fast-paced balls at this distance can be more difficult to counter.

- **Poach:** This is when you cross the center line on the court and hit a ball that would generally be hit by your partner. You would use this shot most often in mixed doubles.
- **Fore- or backhand roll:** As I mentioned earlier, this is one of my best shots in pickleball. It's a volley hit with a forehand topspin at the kitchen line. This drives the ball back at your opponents and prevents them from progressing forward. It also can be a great setup shot for a put-away if the player returning the ball plops it upward. A backhand roll is the same concept, except you simply use your backhand to generate topspin.

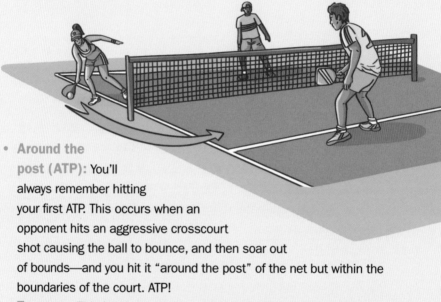

- **Around the post (ATP):** You'll always remember hitting your first ATP. This occurs when an opponent hits an aggressive crosscourt shot causing the ball to bounce, and then soar out of bounds—and you hit it "around the post" of the net but within the boundaries of the court. ATP!
- **Tweener:** This is when you hit a ball between your legs. This shot is mostly used to retrieve lobs you don't have time to properly position yourself to hit.
- **Erne:** This is a shot you hit from the non-volley zone while you jump around the kitchen line. The key is to make sure your feet do not land in the kitchen and that your paddle also doesn't touch the net. You set up this shot when your opponent dinks the ball down the line to you. Ernes are very difficult to defend, as the ball is hit downward

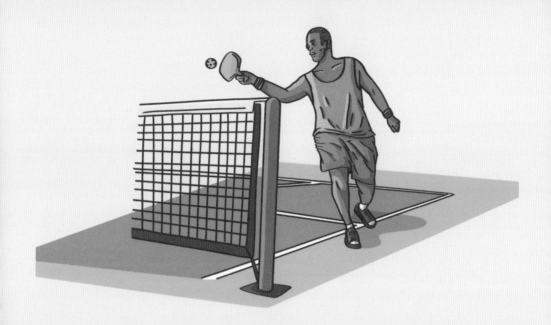

toward your opponent's feet. Pickleball pro Dekel Bar is the CEO of erne shots. He reminds me of a very large gazelle whenever he attempts one.

- **Bert:** An erne you hit in front of your partner. It's basically the same as poaching, but your partner can't get mad because you looked so cool doing it.

***

Now that you know the basic rules of pickleball, you'll soon be fully invested in the sport. Take it from me, I can count on one hand the players I've met who stopped playing pickleball after they started. There really should be a scientific study on how it affects the brain.

Your next stop on your pickleball journey is the magical world of recreational play, where you'll be spending most of your time. Unless, of course, you're just a pickleball prodigy and don't even need to practice before competing in tournaments. I've never met one of those, but anything is possible.

THE TOURNAMENT LIFE

You've been practicing for countless hours, drilling consistently, and are now feeling more confident on the court. The next logical step is to sign up for your first pickleball tournament! From formats and brackets, to finding a partner, this section is chock-full of everything you need to know to register for your first tournament.

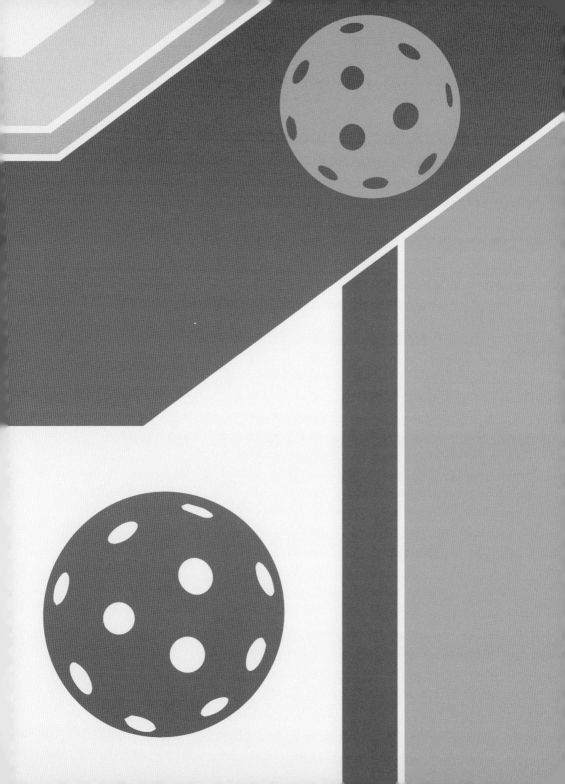

THE MAGICAL WORLD OF TOURNAMENTS

Tournaments might be my favorite thing in all of pickleballdom, and I've played in a lot of them, both big (1,800 registered players) and small (20 registered players). The fans, the players, the vendors, the matches—for a lot of pickleball players, it's as magical as a trip to Disneyland, and the similarities are uncanny.

Instead of a meet-and-greet with Mickey Mouse, you get one with Collin Johns; instead of queuing for a ride, you wait in line for your next court; and instead of a firework finale, you get a gold-medal match on a championship court. Okay, maybe the Disneyland comparison is a bit of a stretch, but attending a pickleball tournament is still tons of fun!

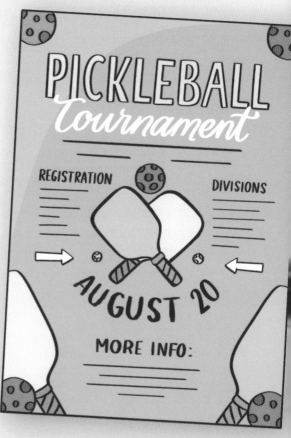

Tournaments give players who might have thought their sports careers were over the opportunity to compete again. It doesn't matter whether you're eighteen or eighty-one, there's a bracket for you to compete in. You'll be playing in a wheelchair? No prob—there's a division for you too. Whether you're at a local or professional tournament, you'll notice many similarities.

When it comes to navigating the registration process, finding a doubles partner, and understanding tournament formats, there's really nowhere you can go to find all of that info in one place. Luckily, I can offer you the benefit of firsthand experience.

WHO SHOULD SIGN UP FOR A TOURNAMENT?

So, how do you know if you're ready to compete in a tournament? As I mentioned previously, the lowest skill level you can be to sign up for many tournaments is 3.0, but some offer 2.0 and 2.5 divisions, as well. If, after reading the common specifications for that level, you feel you're qualified, you can sign up at any time!

It's true! There are really only two requirements to sign up for a tournament:

1. You play pickleball.
2. You have a paddle.

That's it! There's really no "right" time or "aha" moment to signal you're ready. Just do it—there are no barriers to entry, and anyone can participate. Playing in tournaments will also help you level up more quickly because you'll be going up against better players all day (well, until you're beaten, of course).

REGISTRATION

One of the most difficult things about a pickleball tournament is usually signing up for the darn thing! Obviously, I'm exaggerating (but not really). Depending on the tournament, you'll either sign up through your club or the director of your local sports park, or via a website, like pickleball.com, usapickleball.org, or pickleballbrackets.com. For the vast majority, you'll sign up at pickleballtournaments.com.

Once you create an account on pickleballtournaments.com, you'll be able to search and register for upcoming tournaments. Please note, however, that some USA Pickleball–sanctioned tournaments require that you have a USA Pickleball membership. Don't panic if you see this—it's fairly simple (and instantaneous) to obtain a member number via the USA Pickleball website.

After you register for a tournament, you'll also be able to add the events in which you'd like to compete, and select your age group and skill level. Some examples of tournament events you might see listed include:

- Pro Singles, Men
- Pro Singles, Women
- Amateur Singles, Men
- Amateur Singles, Women
- Senior Pro Singles, Men
- Senior Pro Singles, Women

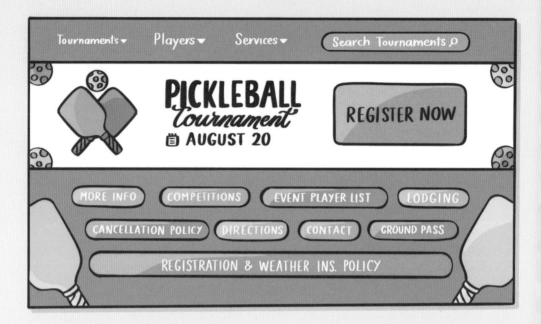

You'll also see men's doubles, women's doubles, and mixed doubles. Some of the less common events include split-age (a team consisting of one pro player and one senior pro player), parapickleball (wheelchair pickleball), and junior events (for ages 18 and under).

In amateur events, there are brackets for the following age groups, with the first three being the most common:

- 19+
- 35+
- 50+
- 60+
- 65+
- 70+
- 85+
- 80+

You'll also need to know your skill level, which I covered previously. For example, say you're twenty-nine years old and a 3.5 skill level; you would sign up for the 19+ age bracket and the 3.5 skill level under the event you wish to play. If you're fifty-two and play at a 4.5 skill level, you would sign up for the 50+ bracket at the 4.5 skill level.

If you're playing doubles, note that you must sign up for the event at the highest skill level on your team. For example, if your partner has a USAPA rating of 4.10, but your skill rating is 3.87, you would have to compete at the 4.0 level. You also have to compete in the age group of your youngest player, so, if your partner is forty-two, but you're twenty-one, you would play in the 19+ age group.

Of course, if you're a pro player (meaning, your skill rating is higher than 5.5), then you're going to want to sign up for pro singles. It's not uncommon to see 5.0+ players in the pro division.

However, I've also seen 4.0- and 4.5-level players sneaking into the pro division in the hopes of playing their favorite pro player. I advise you *not* to do this, if, for no other reason, out of respect. The largest skill jump in pickleball is between levels 5.0 and pro. Even true 5.0-level players struggle to compete with some of the top pros.

Say you were on the Los Angeles Lakers basketball team and had been training for hours every day to condition and prep your body for your next pro game. Imagine showing up expecting to play another pro team, only to find the UCLA college team on the court. It would be confusing and pretty pointless, right? No doubt, the Lakers would win by a landslide, and UCLA would just spend the entire game frustrated because they were unable to compete at that skill level.

I once asked some of my pro friends how they handled these situations, and if they ever enjoyed playing against those who were "playing up." I also asked if they ever took it easy on the lower-level opposing team. The answers varied.

One person said they wouldn't alter their game in any way and would play the same as they would against any professional team. Another said they would use it as a "warm-up" game. However, one thing everyone agreed on was they didn't enjoy playing lower-level teams in the first round. Not only does it make their day feel longer, but it also doesn't feel like a fair match.

PICKLE POINTER

For the best possible tournament experience, always play at your appropriate skill level.

This situation also happens in reverse, though, with higher-level players signing up for lower-level events. This is called "sandbagging," and it's probably the one thing the pickleball community as a whole cannot stand.

You'll usually run into sandbaggers at regional and USA Pickleball National Champion qualifier tournaments because a gold medal in your division is required to get a "golden ticket" to play in the USA Pickleball National Championships at the end of the year. Obviously, intentionally "playing down" to win a gold medal is cheating. It's both unfair and unethical.

PICKLE POINTER

Avoid signing up for a national-qualifier event if it's your first tournament. You'll likely have a lot more fun in a more casual playing environment.

All you have to do to avoid all of this unpleasantness is always play at your appropriate skill level. If you're unsure what that is, ask your local pickleball coach, director, or a club professional for an evaluation so you can find out at what level you should register.

Due to the competitive nature of National qualifier tournaments, I don't recommend you play in one for your first tournament. However, if you ever do sign up for one, you should absolutely do so at your given USA Pickleball Tournament Player Rating (UTPR). Your rating can be found under your player profile at usapickleball.org after you register for a USA Pickleball membership.

During the registration process, there might also be an option to purchase "weather insurance." While most major tournaments take place at venues in warmer climates during the fall and winter, there's never a guarantee when you're dealing with Mother Nature.

One spring, I signed up to play in a tournament in St. George, Utah. When I checked the weather forecast a few days out, it was sunny and clear, so I packed for warmer temperatures. Yeah, turns out, it snowed. Women's doubles day was canceled, and my partner flew in and had to immediately fly back out. It was a sad (and expensive) day.

PICKLE POINTER

Always purchase weather insurance for tournaments in locations with unpredictable weather.

SELECTING A DOUBLES PARTNER

If you'll be playing doubles, it's not usually required that you already have a partner when you register for a tournament. Some players have the same partner for an entire year (this is more common on pro tours) or longer, while others change partners every tournament.

When selecting a partner, you want to make sure you choose someone whose playing style complements yours, as this is critical to perform well at the tournament. You also want someone whose personality meshes well with yours. Your ideal partner might be a friend or family member, but there's one person I'd advise you to avoid partnering with, and that's your significant other.

The most common problem couples face when they also partner up in pickleball is that there's no filter (or, at least, less of one) when it comes to what you say to each other. After all, you likely feel free enough to say all kinds of things to your romantic partner that you would never say to anyone else, and it would be no different during a game of pickleball. Most couples aren't afraid to tell each other exactly what they think of each other's performance between points, and the delivery isn't always in the most encouraging of tones.

Below are just a few things I've overheard couples say to one another during a tournament match:

- "If you're going to take my ball, at least make it over the net."
- "How did you miss that shot? Are you not watching the ball?"
- "All you need to do is get the ball over the net."
- "Say one more word and you're sleeping on the couch tonight."

And that list could go on for pages. If, after reading all of that, you still decide to play mixed doubles with your sig other, I'd keep the number of a marriage counselor handy. Of course, there are always exceptions: Lucy Kovalova and Matt Wright have been playing together (and "together") for years, and they're one of the top mixed-doubles teams in the world.

Your ideal pickleball tournament partner should be someone who is encouraging, uplifting, and fun on the court. Tournaments can be stressful for most people due to the high amount of pressure; you're going to want to be there with someone you vibe well with, both on and off the court.

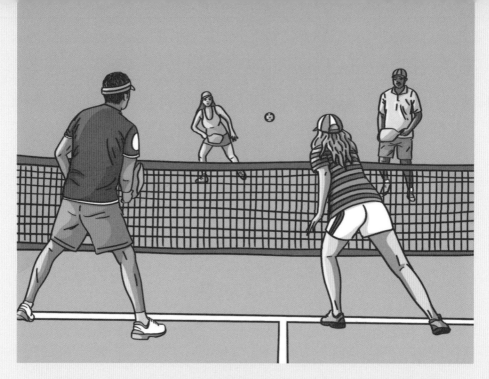

One of my all-time favorite tournament partners was my friend Shea. We had never played a tournament together before, and it was also my first time playing 5.0, 19+, mixed doubles. During one of our matches, I missed a routine forehand dink and immediately apologized. He just smiled and said, "Why are you apologizing? It's not like you purposely hit that dink into the net. Let's have fun!" This set the tone for the remainder of the day, and I felt much more confident on the court afterward.

While we all want a skilled pickleball partner, the most important thing is that their playing style complements yours without compromising any fun. Obviously, in a tournament setting, things can sometimes get heated. Close matches can cause all of us to feel the tension and pressure. It can also cause people to say things they wouldn't normally say to one another. If it's 10–10 and your partner's screaming at you, that's usually when unforced errors occur.

Of course, before signing up to play a tournament together, you're going to want to play some recreational games with anyone you're considering as a possible tournament partner. When you do decide on someone, the best thing you can do for both of you is communicate what you need from a partner and ask what they need from you. (Sounds like couples therapy, doesn't it?)

Because I'm an amateur player who travels the US to play pickleball, I don't always know who my partner will be at all the tournaments I attend. This is called a "blind date," and I'm the CEO of them! When you register on a tournament website, there's usually a section called Player Needing Partners, where all the registered players who didn't sign up with a partner will be listed. Next to their name, you should also see the event(s) for which they need a partner. If you see someone who might be a good fit, you can message them directly from the list.

Unsure how to ask someone to be your blind-date partner? Here's a message I've received from a potential partner:

> Hi,
> I'm looking for a partner in WD (women's doubles) 3.5, 19+ for the PPA Mesa Grand Slam Qualifier. Are you interested in playing together? Would you let me know either way?

I like this message because it covers all the details, and it's short and sweet. It lists the tournament name, skill level, age group, isn't pushy, and asks for a follow-up. Ultimately, I did end up partnering with this person, but even if I'd decided not to, I would have let them know as a courtesy. Don't be a rotten pickle.

Let's look at another example of a good blind-date message:

> Hello,
> I see you are looking for a women's partner for Red Rock. If you are interested in partnering, please let me know. Here are some things about me: I'm 46 years old, I'm rated 3.5, but playing at 4.0 level. I live in the Seattle area and play often. I medaled a few times in 3.5, most recently at the PPA Grand Slam Qualifier (Bronze). I am well rounded and specifically looking for someone who likes the strategic drop-and-dink game.

I like how this person mentioned what they're looking for in a partner and also gave a short pickleball resume. Plus, because this person had played tournaments before, I knew they knew what to expect and could play in a competitive setting.

In case you were wondering, here's an example of a message from someone you *would not* want to partner with:

> Hi,
> Still looking for a mixed doubles partner. Plz text me.

I would *only* accept an offer like this if you're really desperate for a partner and willing to play in any event. Here's another great big no:

> Hello,
> Are you still needing a women's doubles partner? I know I'd have to play down in age. If you could play down at 3.5, that would be great too.

Ideally, you want to play with someone in the same age bracket as you, but that's not mandatory. Asking someone to "play down" at a lower skill level than what they've signed up for, however, would be considered sandbagging (cheating), which is *not* ideal.

The obvious downside of playing with a blind date is you won't know your partner's playing style prior to the tournament; you'll have to figure it out as you're competing. This is why, if you ever do have to play with a blind date, I recommend you both plan to arrive at the tournament venue a day or two early if possible. This way, you can play a recreational game or two and learn more about each other's strengths and weaknesses.

Some important things you'll want to ask anyone you're considering partnering up with include:

- "Do you prefer the left or right side?"
- "Are you comfortable with me taking the middle more?"
- "Are there certain shots you struggle with?"
- "Which shots would you say are your strengths?"

Like any partnership, the biggest asset you'll have on the court is proper communication, and this goes double for blind-date partners.

TOURNAMENT FORMATS

When you browse a pickleball tournament website, you'll see many different kinds of tournaments, but they all fall under one of two categories: sanctioned or unsanctioned. A sanctioned tournament follows USAPA rules, and depending on how well you do, it will affect your UTPR skill-level rating. In a nutshell, if you beat a team that has a higher skill level than you, your rating will go up. If you lose to a team that has a lower skill rating than you, your rating will go down.

A tournament sponsored by Dynamic Universal Pickleball Rating (DUPR) will typically follow USA Pickleball rules, but the outcomes will only affect your DUPR rating.

DOUBLE ELIMINATION

Most major sanctioned tournaments are going to be a double-elimination format. This requires that six or more teams compete in your event, and the seeding of the bracket is based off rating. Seedings are used by the tournament directors to separate the top players in a draw, so they don't play against each other in the early rounds of a tournament. The top seeds in the draw are determined by their current USA Pickleball or DUPR rating.

For the first match, two teams will battle it out in a match of three games, with the best of two out of three winning. Each game is played to 11 points, but a win must be by 2 points. If your team wins, you move to the next part of the draw, while the losing team drops down to the back draw, which is more commonly referred to as the loser's bracket. Now, I prefer to call the latter the "opportunity bracket" because not only is that more optimistic, but it *can* also mean you're just taking the scenic route to the gold-medal match; I'll explain.

In the opportunity bracket (wink), a match consists of one game to 15 points, with a win by 2 points.

If you go on a run—a momentum shift in the game when a team wins a series of points in a row—this could be quite beneficial for your team.

DOUBLE-ELIMINATION FLOWCHART

WINNER'S BRACKET

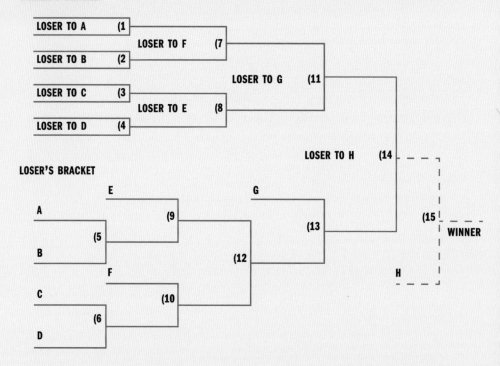

Depending on the tournament, you might even come out of the opportunity bracket and play for the gold medal.

In this case, a gold-medal match would consist of four potential games. First, you'd have to beat the opposing team two out of three games, again, played to 11 points with a win by 2. If your team wins two games, you must play another game to 15 points with a win by 2. If you win this game, congratulations! This is called double-dipping and you are now a gold medalist.

Speaking from experience, this format is especially beneficial for those who aren't early risers and have an early tournament start time. There's just something unappealing about someone screaming, "Come on!" at you at 8 a.m., followed by a series of fast-paced balls flying at your face. But once the caffeine kicks in, it's go-time!

UNSANCTIONED TOURNAMENTS

An unsanctioned tournament is any tournament that isn't USA Pickleball–affiliated. This also means your performance in these won't affect your UTPR rating, which is fantastic if you don't perform well that day.

Likewise, unsanctioned tournaments do not have to follow USA Pickleball rules, but the vast majority of them still do. There are also no referee requirements, but some unsanctioned tournaments still have them for bronze- and gold-medal matches. I highly recommend you play in some unsanctioned tournaments first. They're an outstanding way to dip your feet into tournaments, without the added pressure of performing well enough to maintain your UTPR.

> ## PICKLE POINTER
>
> An unsanctioned tournament is an excellent "trial run" of the tournament experience. You get all the same fun, but without the added pressure of maintaining your UTPR.

ROUND ROBINS

A tournament format you'll run into less often, especially at the larger events, is a round robin—but they're my favorite. These can be either sanctioned or unsanctioned. If your bracket has fewer than six teams, the tournament director may decide to combine yours with another bracket to play a double-elimination or a round-robin format.

In a round robin, each team plays each other once in a match for the best of two out of three games. The games are played to 11 points, and the winning team must win by 2. In some cases, only one game is played to 15 or 21 points, again with a win by 2 points.

After all the teams have played each other once, the winner is determined by the number of matches won. In the event of a tie, those two teams go head-to-head. The team that wins that game gets the higher placement. If three or more teams tie, they're ranked by the total number of games or points won. The larger the number of games won within the group, the higher the overall placement for that team.

What to Do If You ARE the Golden Ticket

It might sound odd, but you can also *be* a golden ticket. I learned this during one of Tyson McGuffin's coaching clinics. At first, I thought it was quite a compliment to be called a "golden ticket." Well, not exactly. *Being* the golden ticket means you're the key to the other team's success because you are the weaker player compared to your partner.

According to McGuffin, if you feel like you're being targeted by the opposing team, then you might be the golden ticket. I have been on more occasions than I'd like to admit, and it's not a pleasant feeling. Your partner will usually be rolling their eyes at you for missing routine shots, while also trying to insert themselves into the point without compromising their lines.

You're trying your best, but every time you send the ball off, it just comes back to you like a boomerang. This is especially true once you get up to the 4.0+ skill levels, where players have decent ball control and singling someone out is a lot more common.

So, what should you do if you're the golden ticket?

First, if you're struggling or starting to feel anxious, call a time-out. As I mentioned previously, you don't get extra credit or anything for not utilizing your time-outs, so use them to devise a plan with your partner. If your game is more consistent on one side than the other, let your partner know.

One strategy you can use is to try stacking with your partner's forehand in the middle, so it's easier for them to take more balls. This will make it much easier for your partner to insert themselves into the point by covering more court. If you return the ball, utilize defensive stacking and switch positions during returns, which might throw off the other team's momentum. Oh, they thought you were only going to be on the right side? Well, your partner's backhand punch is there now, and it's deadly!

If you need your partner to take more balls, make sure you communicate this throughout the point by calling "You!" or "Me!" to avoid any confusion. Sometimes, it might be your partner that's being singled out. This is the time to be that supportive teammate you know you can be. Eye-rolling, groaning, and/or dead silence will only make your partner feel more anxious and uncomfortable. Do your best to be encouraging and praise them on their longer rallies or great shots—this can help boost their confidence *and* their game.

Always remain engaged in the point. The ball can speed up at any time and you have to be ready for it. So, keep that paddle up and stay focused, and there just might be a gold medal in your future!

The round-robin format offers some advantages over the traditional double elimination, one of which is it allows more matches for players. Also, if you're playing with a new or blind-date partner, a round robin will give you some time to get used to each other's playing styles without having to worry about going to the loser's bracket after just one loss. As I mentioned previously, playing with a brand-new partner has some disadvantages in a tournament setting, but a round robin will at least allow you to play several matches. Then, even if the partner chemistry isn't there, the day won't feel like a total waste.

A round robin also rewards the team with the most consistency, which is what makes a good athlete a *great* one. If your team is consistent throughout the day, chances are you'll medal if all the teams are within the same skill-rating range. Unfortunately, consistency won't be the breadwinner if a team is playing down a skill level; that's just a tournament party foul.

GOLDEN TICKETS

If you've ever seen the movie *Willy Wonka and the Chocolate Factory*, you'll remember the "golden tickets" the children found in their chocolate bars, which earned them a once-in-a-lifetime tour of Willy's Chocolate Factory.

In pickleball, there are, in fact, numerous types of golden tickets, but the most coveted is USA Pickleball Nationals. This is, by far, one of the most prestigious pickleball tournaments of the year, and if you're an amateur who has a passion for pickleball, it might be your top goal to compete here. It's important to note, however, that not just anyone with decent pickleball skills can compete at Nationals, and golden tickets aren't something that are easily attained.

In fact, some might argue they're even more difficult to get than Willy Wonka's! To compete at Nationals, you first have to win a gold medal in your event at one of the many qualifier tournaments held throughout the US. You must also win a gold medal in every event in which you want to compete at Nationals. For example, if you won a gold medal in men's doubles and singles, you could compete in men's doubles and singles at Nationals, but not in mixed doubles.

If you don't win a golden ticket at some point during the year, the tournament also holds a lottery and players are selected at random to register. This is a great option for those who don't live near one of the many national qualifier tournaments, but would still like to compete.

One thing to note when you're signing up for a national qualifier tournament is that people will typically play at the lowest level they can. This is because the tournament pulls players based on their USA Pickleball Tournament Player Rating (UTPR), which is generally lower than their true skill level. This means you can expect a higher level of play even at the lower levels (remember when we talked about sandbagging?).

Once upon a pickle star, I signed up for a national qualifier tournament at my home club in Newport Beach, California. I was a 3.5 skill-level player who thought she was a lot better than she actually was, and I signed up for both 3.5 women's and mixed doubles in the hope of securing a golden ticket.

I was confident at the time that I was a sandbagger, and it would be an easy win for me and my partner. Well, I got served a fat slice of humble pie that weekend. I don't believe I won any matches at all. As a matter of fact, I don't even think any of them were close. It was quite humiliating and I was very embarrassed.

By the end of that tournament weekend, I learned that I was playing teams ranging from 4.0 to 5.0 skill levels in the 3.5 division. Is that fair? Well, no. However, short of fixing the current UTPR rating system, there's really no way to rectify this.

The moral of the story is if you plan to sign up for a national qualifier tournament, don't be surprised if you're playing against teams that are a higher skill level than yours. I'd also advise against making a national qualifier your first tournament; they're absolutely a lot of fun, but there are so many other tournament options out there that are a lot more casual.

* * *

Once you've signed up for your first tournament and have taken a moment to celebrate (go you!), it's time to start prepping to win.

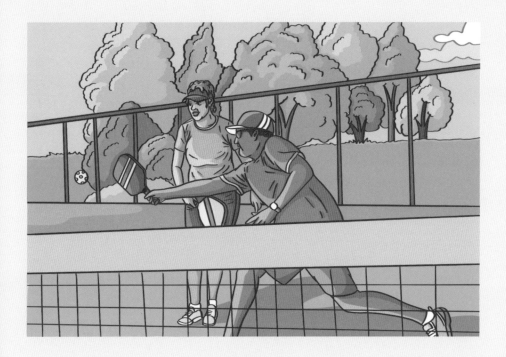

PREPPING YOUR BODY TO PLAY

Putting yourself in the right mindset to play pickleball is the first step in crafting a winning game strategy, but getting your body prepared to play is just as, if not more, important. Hitting the court cold is a recipe for disaster, so in addition to being constantly hydrated, you must take the time to stretch and do other warm-up activities. To keep your body in ready-to-play mode, do these exercises every day if you can, not just before a match.

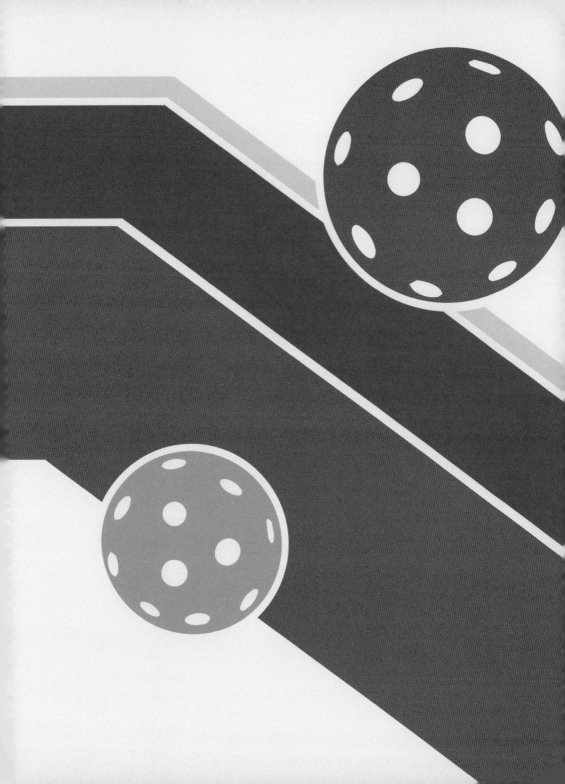

No one wants to pull a muscle during the first round of a tournament and have to forfeit. That's why the first thing you should do before stepping on a court is stretch. A year after I started playing pickleball, I began seeing a doctor who advised I try dynamic neural adaptive training to help me keep any anxiety at bay and stay focused on the court. He also helped me create a dynamic stretching routine. Dynamic stretches slowly loosen your muscles and lubricate your joints.

If I'm feeling a bit anxious, I also put in my earbuds and listen to some music while I go through my routine to help me relax.

Below is the routine I always go through before a tournament match, and it only takes about ten minutes to complete. For standing exercises, start at or near the net and return when you reach the baseline:

1. **Slow-paced jog forward and backward:** This is just what it sounds like—you jog forward slowly. You'll need around 25 yards (23 m) of space to perform your jogs forward and backward. When you reach the end of your allotted space jogging forward, start jogging backward (be careful not to trip over anything). Repeat twice.

2. **Low side shuffle:** Start in a squat position, and then, leading with your right leg, "shuffle" to the right, and then to the left. Repeat twice.

3. **Zombie walk:** Start in a standing position, swing one leg forward, and then try to touch your toes. Repeat each leg twice.

4. **Karaoke runs:** Start in a standing position with your arms bent and held near your head. Cross your left leg over your right. Step out of the pose with your right leg, and then twist your left leg behind you. Step with your left again, but this time, end with a kick. Then, come back starting on your right leg. Watch this one on YouTube a few times to get the hang of it.

> ## PICKLE POINTER
>
> You can follow any routine you want, but make sure you always stretch properly before a tournament. There's nothing worse than having to push through with sore muscles when you still have hours left to play.

5. **Tall-march stretch:** Jump vertically with one knee about hip height, and then reach overhead with one arm.

6. **Cross-march stretch:** Same as the tall-march stretch, but this time, cross your knee toward the opposite hand, and then repeat with the opposite knee.

7. **Iron-cross stretch:** Lie on your back on your towel and extend your arms out to your sides. Raise your right leg straight up, and then rotate your hips to the left until your right leg touchs the ground. Hold for five seconds, and then repeat on the other side. Repeat five times on each side.

8. **Leg-crossover sphinx stretch:** Lie on your stomach on your towel with your forehead touching the floor. Brace yourself with your forearms as you slowly raise your shoulders and upper body. Slowly cross your right leg over your left, until your right toes touch the floor. Return to center and repeat with the left leg. Do five reps on each leg.

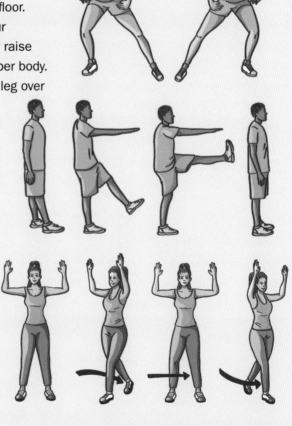

After you complete your stretching routine, it's time to hydrate and then head to your court with your partner to warm up.

WARMING UP

When you arrive at your court, place your bags somewhere safe nearby, but off-court, so you won't trip over anything mid-match. When bags are too close to the court, they could also interfere with ATPs or ernes. Once, as I was warming up before a match, someone on the opposing team asked the referee to tell me to move my bag off the court because she needed that space for ATPs. She actually didn't ATP once during that match and my bag got all muddy. I was pretty annoyed, but safety first!

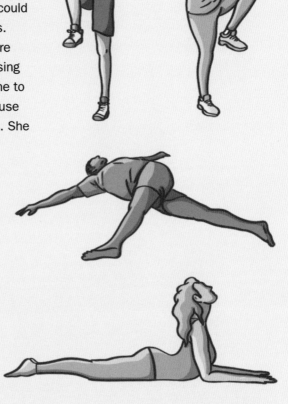

If your match has a referee, before you warm up, they will ask all players to come in for a paddle check. They'll be looking to make sure all of them have a USAPA-approved sticker or label. If you're playing in an unsanctioned tournament and don't have a referee, your paddle will most likely not be checked unless deemed necessary by the tournament director.

The list of approved paddles is constantly changing, so be sure to check the USA Pickleball website before any tournament to see the most current list. A ref might also touch the surface of your paddle to see if it's been altered in any way.

While you warm up, the opposing team will be doing the same right next to you. This is a great opportunity to observe and see if there are any shots at which either of them is inconsistent. You can also note any strengths they might have, such as a low, aggressive drive or a forehand dink with a lot of topspin.

One of the biggest mistakes you can make is underestimating your opponents based on their appearance. That old adage "don't judge a book by its cover" applies in pickleball, as well, and I've been on both sides of this coin. Often, when people see blonde me, dressed in pink, walking to their court, they automatically assume I'm a terrible player. Of course, they quickly find out I'm no beginner. Numerous times, I've also been embarrassed on the court by people more than twice my age. That's part of the beauty of pickleball.

Depending on how tight the tournament's schedule is, you'll usually be allowed anywhere from two to five minutes to warm up with your partner before a match. If there's a referee, they will be timing you. This is the main reason you want to get to a tournament early—that warm-up time is precious!

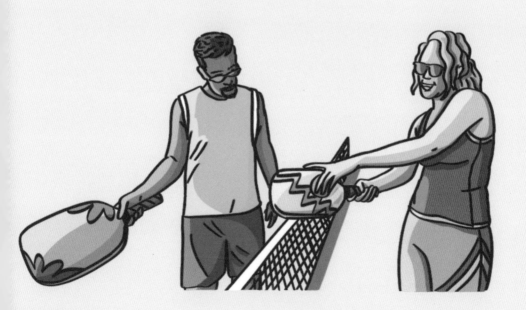

GLOSSARY

Ace: A serve that is not returned by the opposing team.

Around the post (ATP): A specialty shot in which you return the pickleball from under the top of the net and around its post.

Back draw: Also known as the "consolation," "losers," or "opportunity" bracket, it's where a team is moved after losing their first match in a tournament.

Backcourt: The few feet at the back of the court near the baseline.

Backhand: A racquet-sport strike in which the back of your dominant hand is facing the direction in which you're hitting the ball.

Backhand roll: A backhand volley hit that generates topspin at the kitchen line.

Backspin: Hitting the ball in a high-to-low motion, causing it to spin backward.

Backswing: The backward movement you make with your arm and paddle before hitting the ball.

Ball on: A player on another court will call this out if a stray pickleball of theirs rolls onto your court.

Baseline: This line is 22 feet (6.7 m) from the net on each side to mark the end of the pickleball court.

Bert: An erne you poach from your partner.

Block shot: Any volley that takes the pace off a drive.

Centerline: The line on the pickleball court that divides the service area in half. It runs from the non-volley zone to the baseline.

Clean winner: When you win a point because the opposing player or team doesn't hit the ball.

Crosscourt dink: When you hit a dink from one corner of the court across the net to the other corner of the court.

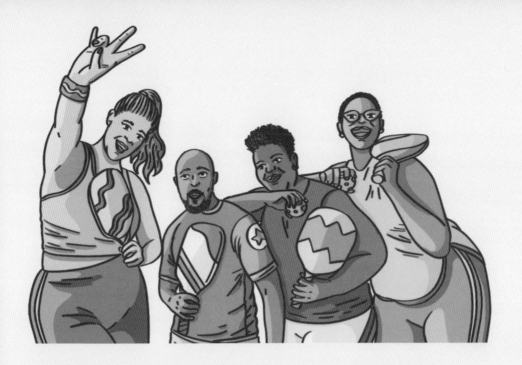

Counterattack: An aggressive return volley shot after an opponent has hit one to you.

Dink: A shot hit at or near the net that is just high enough to go over, but low enough that it can't be hit from the air by the opposition.

Double hit: When the ball hits your paddle twice in one continuous ground stroke.

Doubles: A match with four players (two on each side of the net).

Down-the-line dink: A dink hit to the player directly in front of you.

Draw: The order in which matches are to be played in a tournament.

Drill: A practice exercise designed to help a player develop or improve a specific skill or set of skills.

Drive: Returning a ground stroke or volley as hard as you can.

Drop serve: A type of serve in which the ball is dropped from shoulder height, allowed to bounce, and then hit diagonally across the court to the receiver.

Erne: Named after Erne Perry, who perfected it, this is a shot hit from the non-volley zone while you jump around the kitchen line.

Foot fault: This occurs if your foot touches the baseline as you're striking the ball, or if either of your feet are touching any part of the perimeter lines surrounding the non-volley zone when you hit a ball out of the air.

Forced error: A shot that causes the other player or team to make an error.

Forehand: A racquet-sport strike in which the palm of your dominant hand is facing the direction in which you're hitting the ball.

Forehand roll: A forehand volley hit that generates topspin at the kitchen line.

Ground stroke: Hitting the ball after it's bounced on the ground.

Half volley: A ground-stroke shot in which the paddle hits the ball immediately after it bounces from the court, but before it reaches its full height.

Hands battle: A series of fast volleys back and forth from the kitchen line between two players or teams.

Hard game: A game in which the ball is being returned hard from the front or back of the court.

Hinder: Anything that interferes with the game and affects play during a point.

The kitchen: Also called the "non-volley zone," this is the area of the court 7 feet (2.1 m) from both sides of the net, and from sideline to sideline.

Kitchen line: The line from sideline to sideline that divides the kitchen from the remainder of the court. Your feet must always be behind this line when volleying.

Let: A serve that hits the net but still lands properly beyond the non-volley zone.

Line call: The decision made as to whether a ball was in- or out-of-bounds.

Lob: A shot hit as high and deep as possible in an attempt to pull a player (or players) away from the kitchen line.

Midcourt: The area of the court between the kitchen line and the baseline.

Mixed doubles: A doubles game with one man and one woman on both sides of the net.

Non-volley zone (NVZ): Also called "the kitchen," it's the 7-foot (2.1 m) area from the net on both sides, and from sideline to sideline. Balls cannot be volleyed when you are standing inside this area.

Overhead smash: A shot in which the paddle starts above the player's head, followed by a downward motion.

Passing shot: A shot that's out of your opponent's reach. Occurs often in singles' matches, but can happen in doubles' matches as well.

Permanent object: An immovable item or structure near the court that could hinder gameplay.

Pickled: Also called a "bagel," this is when a team scores zero points in a pickleball game.

Poach: When your doubles' partner crosses over to your side of the court to hit a shot.

Punch: A quick, minimal-backswing volley used as an aggressive attack.

Put-away: A shot that is extremely difficult for the opposing team to return.

Rally: A point that's played out from the moment the ball is served until there's a fault.

Rally scoring: In this type of scoring, the team that wins the point gets it regardless of who served the ball. The team who wins the point also gains the right to serve.

Reflex volley: When a player receiving the ball has no time to react and instinctively hits a volley to defend.

Reset: Any shot that drops the ball in the kitchen.

Rubber match: Also known as the "tie-breaker" match, it's the game played after one team wins the first game and the other team wins the second and a third game is played as the tie-breaker.

Run: A series of points won consecutively by the serving team.

Seed: Your (or your team's) ranking among other teams in your draw in a tournament.

Serve: Using an underhand paddle stroke to hit the pickleball and begin a game. You must serve from behind the baseline, and on the left or right side of the centerline.

Server number: The number (1 or 2) each player on a doubles team receives to designate the order in which they will serve.

Service area: Also called the service "box" or "court," this is the area on either side of the centerline beyond the non-volley zone.

Service let: A serve that hits the net cord and lands in the service area.

Sideline: The lines on each side of the court that are perpendicular to the net.

Side-out: When the serving player or team loses the serve and the ball is given to the other player or team.

Singles: A game between two players, with one on each side of the net, and only one serve per side-out.

Skinny singles: A game of singles during which only half of the court is used.

Slice: A ground stroke or volley hit with backspin.

Soft game: A game in which the ball is returned softly into the non-volley zone.

Spin serve: Spinning the ball in one or both hands before an underhand serve.

Switch: When you signal your partner to retrieve a lob on your side of the court, and then you switch sides.

Tagging: Also called a "body bag" or "peg," this is when you intentionally hit an opposing player's body with the pickleball to win a point.

Third shot: Each point in pickleball usually follows a three-shot sequence: the serve, return, and this shot hit by the serving team.

Topspin: When you hit the ball from low to high, causing it to spin forward in the direction it's traveling.

Tweener: Hitting a ball between your legs.

Underhand: A stroke in which the paddle is traveling in an upward motion to hit the ball. You must serve underhand in pickleball.

Unforced error: When a player makes a mistake or commits a fault on a return shot.

Volley: When a ball is hit in the air before it hits the ground during a rally. You can only volley if the ball has bounced once in each team's court.

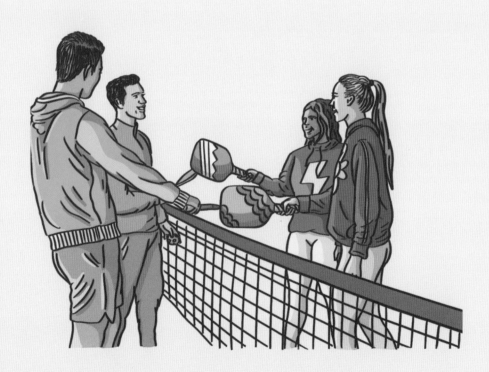

TRACK YOUR PROGRESS

Taking note of your stats is a valuable practice in any sport. It helps you see how fast or slow you are improving and assists in making meaningful goals to aim for in the future. In the following pages you can keep track of all the details of your games, how your skills and gameplay are developing, your training, and any long-term planning that will help you become a better pickleball player.

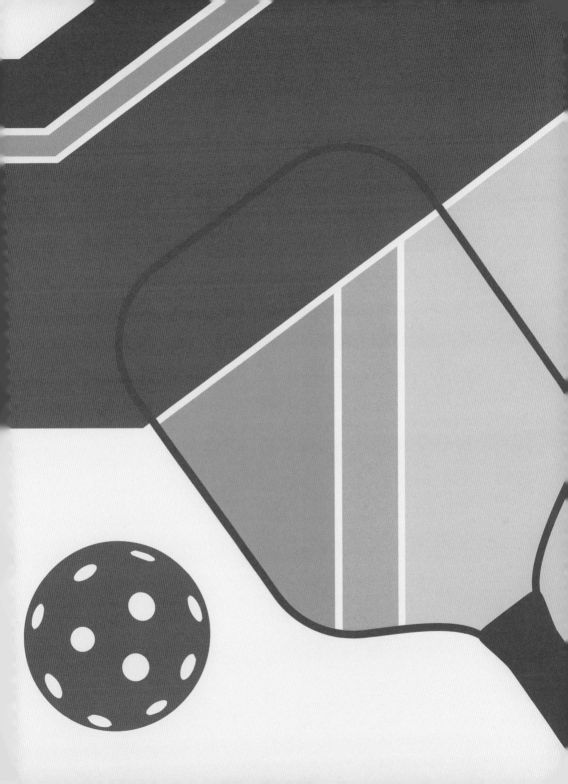

PICKLEBALL PLANNER

Month _____ **Week** _____

Date _____
Location _____
Players _____
_____
Scores _____ _____ _____

Date _____
Location _____
Players _____
_____
Scores _____ _____ _____

Date _____
Location _____
Players _____
_____
Scores _____ _____ _____

Date _____
Location _____
Players _____
_____
Scores _____ _____ _____

Date _____
Location _____
Players _____
_____
Scores _____ _____ _____

Date _____
Location _____
Players _____
_____
Scores _____ _____ _____

Date _____
Location _____
Players _____
_____
Scores _____ _____ _____

Date _____
Location _____
Players _____
_____
Scores _____ _____ _____

Things to improve on:

Player notes:

PICKLEBALL PLANNER

Month _____ Week _____

Date _____
Location _____
Players _____
_____
Scores _____ _____ _____

Date _____
Location _____
Players _____
_____
Scores _____ _____ _____

Date _____
Location _____
Players _____
_____
Scores _____ _____ _____

Date _____
Location _____
Players _____
_____
Scores _____ _____ _____

Date _____
Location _____
Players _____
_____
Scores _____ _____ _____

Date _____
Location _____
Players _____
_____
Scores _____ _____ _____

Date _____
Location _____
Players _____
_____
Scores _____ _____ _____

Date _____
Location _____
Players _____
_____
Scores _____ _____ _____

Things to improve on:

Player notes:

PICKLEBALL PLANNER

Month _____ **Week** _____

Date _____
Location _____
Players _____
_____
Scores _____ _____ _____

Date _____
Location _____
Players _____
_____
Scores _____ _____ _____

Date _____
Location _____
Players _____
_____
Scores _____ _____ _____

Date _____
Location _____
Players _____
_____
Scores _____ _____ _____

Date _____
Location _____
Players _____
_____
Scores _____ _____ _____

Date _____
Location _____
Players _____
_____
Scores _____ _____ _____

Date _____
Location _____
Players _____
_____
Scores _____ _____ _____

Date _____
Location _____
Players _____
_____
Scores _____ _____ _____

Things to improve on:

Player notes:

PICKLEBALL PLANNER

Month _____ Week _____

Date _____
Location _____
Players _____
_____
Scores _____ _____ _____

Date _____
Location _____
Players _____
_____
Scores _____ _____ _____

Date _____
Location _____
Players _____
_____
Scores _____ _____ _____

Date _____
Location _____
Players _____
_____
Scores _____ _____ _____

Date _____
Location _____
Players _____
_____
Scores _____ _____ _____

Date _____
Location _____
Players _____
_____
Scores _____ _____ _____

Date _____
Location _____
Players _____
_____
Scores _____ _____ _____

Date _____
Location _____
Players _____
_____
Scores _____ _____ _____

Things to improve on:

Player notes:

SKILLS ASSESSMENT

SKILLS	1	2	3	4	5
SERVE					
RETURN					
3RD SHOT DRIVE					
TRANSITION ZONE					
DIGS					
BLOCKING					
DINKING					
VOLLEYS					
ATTACK					
LOB					
LOB DEFENSE					
CONSISTENCY					

KEY: **1** Not Present **2** Needs Development **3** OK **4** Good **5** Great

OBSERVE & ANALYZE

	Never	Less Often	Often	Always
Do you move the opponent to the side?				
Do you move the opponent back and forth?				
Do you give yourself enough time to get to the kitchen line when you return the serve?				
Do you demonstrate a variety of serves?				
Do you select shots appropriately?				
Do you hit into open areas of the court?				
Do you try to attack the ball at the first available opportunity?				
Do you play to the opposition's weakness?				
Do you control the point?				

What are my strengths in the gameplay areas listed above?

What are my weaknesses in the gameplay areas listed above?

How can I improve on my strengths and weaknesses in the gameplay areas listed above?

PICKLEBALL TRAINING

- [ ] Warm up/Dynamic stretching
- [ ] Cardio
- [ ] Strength training
- [ ] Drills
- [ ] Recreational play
- [ ] Semi-competitive play
- [ ] Competitive play
- [ ] Tournament play
- [ ] Cool down/Static stretching

NOTES

LONG-TERM GOALS

PICKLEBALL PLANNER

Month _____ **Week** _____

Date _____
Location _____
Players _____
_____
Scores _____ _____ _____

Date _____
Location _____
Players _____
_____
Scores _____ _____ _____

Date _____
Location _____
Players _____
_____
Scores _____ _____ _____

Date _____
Location _____
Players _____
_____
Scores _____ _____ _____

Date _____
Location _____
Players _____
_____
Scores _____ _____ _____

Date _____
Location _____
Players _____
_____
Scores _____ _____ _____

Date _____
Location _____
Players _____
_____
Scores _____ _____ _____

Date _____
Location _____
Players _____
_____
Scores _____ _____ _____

Things to improve on:

Player notes:

PICKLEBALL PLANNER

Month _____ Week _____

Date _____
Location _____
Players _____
_____
Scores _____ _____ _____

Date _____
Location _____
Players _____
_____
Scores _____ _____ _____

Date _____
Location _____
Players _____
_____
Scores _____ _____ _____

Date _____
Location _____
Players _____
_____
Scores _____ _____ _____

Date _____
Location _____
Players _____
_____
Scores _____ _____ _____

Date _____
Location _____
Players _____
_____
Scores _____ _____ _____

Date _____
Location _____
Players _____
_____
Scores _____ _____ _____

Date _____
Location _____
Players _____
_____
Scores _____ _____ _____

Things to improve on:

Player notes:

PICKLEBALL PLANNER

Month _____ **Week** _____

Date _____
Location _____
Players _____
_____
Scores _____ _____ _____

Date _____
Location _____
Players _____
_____
Scores _____ _____ _____

Date _____
Location _____
Players _____
_____
Scores _____ _____ _____

Date _____
Location _____
Players _____
_____
Scores _____ _____ _____

Date _____
Location _____
Players _____
_____
Scores _____ _____ _____

Date _____
Location _____
Players _____
_____
Scores _____ _____ _____

Date _____
Location _____
Players _____
_____
Scores _____ _____ _____

Date _____
Location _____
Players _____
_____
Scores _____ _____ _____

Things to improve on:

Player notes:

PICKLEBALL PLANNER

Month _____ Week _____

Date _____
Location _____
Players _____
_____
Scores _____ _____ _____

Date _____
Location _____
Players _____
_____
Scores _____ _____ _____

Date _____
Location _____
Players _____
_____
Scores _____ _____ _____

Date _____
Location _____
Players _____
_____
Scores _____ _____ _____

Date _____
Location _____
Players _____
_____
Scores _____ _____ _____

Date _____
Location _____
Players _____
_____
Scores _____ _____ _____

Date _____
Location _____
Players _____
_____
Scores _____ _____ _____

Date _____
Location _____
Players _____
_____
Scores _____ _____ _____

Things to improve on:

Player notes:

SKILLS ASSESSMENT

SKILLS	1	2	3	4	5
SERVE					
RETURN					
3RD SHOT DRIVE					
TRANSITION ZONE					
DIGS					
BLOCKING					
DINKING					
VOLLEYS					
ATTACK					
LOB					
LOB DEFENSE					
CONSISTENCY					

KEY: **1** Not Present **2** Needs Development **3** OK **4** Good **5** Great

OBSERVE & ANALYZE

	Never	Less Often	Often	Always
Do you move the opponent to the side?				
Do you move the opponent back and forth?				
Do you give yourself enough time to get to the kitchen line when you return the serve?				
Do you demonstrate a variety of serves?				
Do you select shots appropriately?				
Do you hit into open areas of the court?				
Do you try to attack the ball at the first available opportunity?				
Do you play to the opposition's weakness?				
Do you control the point?				

What are my strengths in the gameplay areas listed above?

What are my weaknesses in the gameplay areas listed above?

How can I improve on my strengths and weaknesses in the gameplay areas listed above?

PICKLEBALL TRAINING

- [ ] Warm up/Dynamic stretching
- [ ] Cardio
- [ ] Strength training
- [ ] Drills
- [ ] Recreational play
- [ ] Semi-competitive play
- [ ] Competitive play
- [ ] Tournament play
- [ ] Cool down/Static stretching

NOTES

LONG-TERM GOALS

PICKLEBALL PLANNER

Month _____ **Week** _____

Date _____
Location _____
Players _____
_____
Scores _____ _____ _____

Date _____
Location _____
Players _____
_____
Scores _____ _____ _____

Date _____
Location _____
Players _____
_____
Scores _____ _____ _____

Date _____
Location _____
Players _____
_____
Scores _____ _____ _____

Date _____
Location _____
Players _____
_____
Scores _____ _____ _____

Date _____
Location _____
Players _____
_____
Scores _____ _____ _____

Date _____
Location _____
Players _____
_____
Scores _____ _____ _____

Date _____
Location _____
Players _____
_____
Scores _____ _____ _____

Things to improve on:

Player notes:

PICKLEBALL PLANNER

Month _____ Week _____

Date _____
Location _____
Players _____
_____
Scores _____ _____ _____

Date _____
Location _____
Players _____
_____
Scores _____ _____ _____

Date _____
Location _____
Players _____
_____
Scores _____ _____ _____

Date _____
Location _____
Players _____
_____
Scores _____ _____ _____

Date _____
Location _____
Players _____
_____
Scores _____ _____ _____

Date _____
Location _____
Players _____
_____
Scores _____ _____ _____

Date _____
Location _____
Players _____
_____
Scores _____ _____ _____

Date _____
Location _____
Players _____
_____
Scores _____ _____ _____

Things to improve on:

Player notes:

PICKLEBALL PLANNER

Month _____ **Week** _____

Date _____
Location _____
Players _____
_____
Scores _____ _____ _____

Date _____
Location _____
Players _____
_____
Scores _____ _____ _____

Date _____
Location _____
Players _____
_____
Scores _____ _____ _____

Date _____
Location _____
Players _____
_____
Scores _____ _____ _____

Date _____
Location _____
Players _____
_____
Scores _____ _____ _____

Date _____
Location _____
Players _____
_____
Scores _____ _____ _____

Date _____
Location _____
Players _____
_____
Scores _____ _____ _____

Date _____
Location _____
Players _____
_____
Scores _____ _____ _____

Things to improve on:

Player notes:

PICKLEBALL PLANNER

Month _____ Week _____

Date _____
Location _____
Players _____
_____
Scores _____ _____ _____

Date _____
Location _____
Players _____
_____
Scores _____ _____ _____

Date _____
Location _____
Players _____
_____
Scores _____ _____ _____

Date _____
Location _____
Players _____
_____
Scores _____ _____ _____

Date _____
Location _____
Players _____
_____
Scores _____ _____ _____

Date _____
Location _____
Players _____
_____
Scores _____ _____ _____

Date _____
Location _____
Players _____
_____
Scores _____ _____ _____

Date _____
Location _____
Players _____
_____
Scores _____ _____ _____

Things to improve on:

Player notes:

SKILLS ASSESSMENT

SKILLS	1	2	3	4	5
SERVE					
RETURN					
3RD SHOT DRIVE					
TRANSITION ZONE					
DIGS					
BLOCKING					
DINKING					
VOLLEYS					
ATTACK					
LOB					
LOB DEFENSE					
CONSISTENCY					

KEY: **1** Not Present   **2** Needs Development   **3** OK   **4** Good   **5** Great

OBSERVE & ANALYZE

	Never	Less Often	Often	Always
Do you move the opponent to the side?				
Do you move the opponent back and forth?				
Do you give yourself enough time to get to the kitchen line when you return the serve?				
Do you demonstrate a variety of serves?				
Do you select shots appropriately?				
Do you hit into open areas of the court?				
Do you try to attack the ball at the first available opportunity?				
Do you play to the opposition's weakness?				
Do you control the point?				

What are my strengths in the gameplay areas listed above?

What are my weaknesses in the gameplay areas listed above?

How can I improve on my strengths and weaknesses in the gameplay areas listed above?

PICKLEBALL TRAINING

- [ ] Warm up/Dynamic stretching
- [ ] Cardio
- [ ] Strength training
- [ ] Drills
- [ ] Recreational play
- [ ] Semi-competitive play
- [ ] Competitive play
- [ ] Tournament play
- [ ] Cool down/Static stretching

NOTES

LONG-TERM GOALS

PICKLEBALL PLANNER

Month _____   **Week** _____

Date _____
Location _____
Players _____
_____
Scores _____ _____ _____

Date _____
Location _____
Players _____
_____
Scores _____ _____ _____

Date _____
Location _____
Players _____
_____
Scores _____ _____ _____

Date _____
Location _____
Players _____
_____
Scores _____ _____ _____

Date _____
Location _____
Players _____
_____
Scores _____ _____ _____

Date _____
Location _____
Players _____
_____
Scores _____ _____ _____

Date _____
Location _____
Players _____
_____
Scores _____ _____ _____

Date _____
Location _____
Players _____
_____
Scores _____ _____ _____

Things to improve on:

Player notes:

PICKLEBALL PLANNER

Month _____ Week _____

Date _____
Location _____
Players _____
_____
Scores _____ _____ _____

Date _____
Location _____
Players _____
_____
Scores _____ _____ _____

Date _____
Location _____
Players _____
_____
Scores _____ _____ _____

Date _____
Location _____
Players _____
_____
Scores _____ _____ _____

Date _____
Location _____
Players _____
_____
Scores _____ _____ _____

Date _____
Location _____
Players _____
_____
Scores _____ _____ _____

Date _____
Location _____
Players _____
_____
Scores _____ _____ _____

Date _____
Location _____
Players _____
_____
Scores _____ _____ _____

Things to improve on:

Player notes:

PICKLEBALL PLANNER

Month _____ **Week** _____

Date _____
Location _____
Players _____
_____
Scores _____ _____ _____

Date _____
Location _____
Players _____
_____
Scores _____ _____ _____

Date _____
Location _____
Players _____
_____
Scores _____ _____ _____

Date _____
Location _____
Players _____
_____
Scores _____ _____ _____

Date _____
Location _____
Players _____
_____
Scores _____ _____ _____

Date _____
Location _____
Players _____
_____
Scores _____ _____ _____

Date _____
Location _____
Players _____
_____
Scores _____ _____ _____

Date _____
Location _____
Players _____
_____
Scores _____ _____ _____

Things to improve on:

Player notes:

PICKLEBALL PLANNER

Month _____ Week _____

Date _____
Location _____
Players _____
_____
Scores _____ _____ _____

Date _____
Location _____
Players _____
_____
Scores _____ _____ _____

Date _____
Location _____
Players _____
_____
Scores _____ _____ _____

Date _____
Location _____
Players _____
_____
Scores _____ _____ _____

Date _____
Location _____
Players _____
_____
Scores _____ _____ _____

Date _____
Location _____
Players _____
_____
Scores _____ _____ _____

Date _____
Location _____
Players _____
_____
Scores _____ _____ _____

Date _____
Location _____
Players _____
_____
Scores _____ _____ _____

Things to improve on:

Player notes:

SKILLS ASSESSMENT

SKILLS	1	2	3	4	5
SERVE					
RETURN					
3RD SHOT DRIVE					
TRANSITION ZONE					
DIGS					
BLOCKING					
DINKING					
VOLLEYS					
ATTACK					
LOB					
LOB DEFENSE					
CONSISTENCY					

KEY: **1** Not Present **2** Needs Development **3** OK **4** Good **5** Great

OBSERVE & ANALYZE

	Never	Less Often	Often	Always
Do you move the opponent to the side?				
Do you move the opponent back and forth?				
Do you give yourself enough time to get to the kitchen line when you return the serve?				
Do you demonstrate a variety of serves?				
Do you select shots appropriately?				
Do you hit into open areas of the court?				
Do you try to attack the ball at the first available opportunity?				
Do you play to the opposition's weakness?				
Do you control the point?				

What are my strengths in the gameplay areas listed above?

What are my weaknesses in the gameplay areas listed above?

How can I improve on my strengths and weaknesses in the gameplay areas listed above?

PICKLEBALL TRAINING

- [ ] Warm up/Dynamic stretching
- [ ] Cardio
- [ ] Strength training
- [ ] Drills
- [ ] Recreational play
- [ ] Semi-competitive play
- [ ] Competitive play
- [ ] Tournament play
- [ ] Cool down/Static stretching

NOTES

LONG-TERM GOALS

PICKLEBALL PLANNER

Month _____ **Week** _____

Date _____
Location _____
Players _____
_____
Scores _____ _____ _____

Date _____
Location _____
Players _____
_____
Scores _____ _____ _____

Date _____
Location _____
Players _____
_____
Scores _____ _____ _____

Date _____
Location _____
Players _____
_____
Scores _____ _____ _____

Date _____
Location _____
Players _____
_____
Scores _____ _____ _____

Date _____
Location _____
Players _____
_____
Scores _____ _____ _____

Date _____
Location _____
Players _____
_____
Scores _____ _____ _____

Date _____
Location _____
Players _____
_____
Scores _____ _____ _____

Things to improve on:

Player notes:

PICKLEBALL PLANNER

Month _____ Week _____

Date _____
Location _____
Players _____
_____
Scores _____ _____ _____

Date _____
Location _____
Players _____
_____
Scores _____ _____ _____

Date _____
Location _____
Players _____
_____
Scores _____ _____ _____

Date _____
Location _____
Players _____
_____
Scores _____ _____ _____

Date _____
Location _____
Players _____
_____
Scores _____ _____ _____

Date _____
Location _____
Players _____
_____
Scores _____ _____ _____

Date _____
Location _____
Players _____
_____
Scores _____ _____ _____

Date _____
Location _____
Players _____
_____
Scores _____ _____ _____

Things to improve on:

Player notes:

PICKLEBALL PLANNER

Month _____ **Week** _____

Date _____
Location _____
Players _____
_____
Scores _____ _____ _____

Date _____
Location _____
Players _____
_____
Scores _____ _____ _____

Date _____
Location _____
Players _____
_____
Scores _____ _____ _____

Date _____
Location _____
Players _____
_____
Scores _____ _____ _____

Date _____
Location _____
Players _____
_____
Scores _____ _____ _____

Date _____
Location _____
Players _____
_____
Scores _____ _____ _____

Date _____
Location _____
Players _____
_____
Scores _____ _____ _____

Date _____
Location _____
Players _____
_____
Scores _____ _____ _____

Things to improve on:

Player notes:

PICKLEBALL PLANNER

Month _____   Week _____

Date _____
Location _____
Players _____
_____
Scores _____ _____ _____

Date _____
Location _____
Players _____
_____
Scores _____ _____ _____

Date _____
Location _____
Players _____
_____
Scores _____ _____ _____

Date _____
Location _____
Players _____
_____
Scores _____ _____ _____

Date _____
Location _____
Players _____
_____
Scores _____ _____ _____

Date _____
Location _____
Players _____
_____
Scores _____ _____ _____

Date _____
Location _____
Players _____
_____
Scores _____ _____ _____

Date _____
Location _____
Players _____
_____
Scores _____ _____ _____

Things to improve on:

Player notes:

SKILLS ASSESSMENT

SKILLS	1	2	3	4	5
SERVE	●	●	●	●	●
RETURN	●	●	●	●	●
3RD SHOT DRIVE	●	●	●	●	●
TRANSITION ZONE	●	●	●	●	●
DIGS	●	●	●	●	●
BLOCKING	●	●	●	●	●
DINKING	●	●	●	●	●
VOLLEYS	●	●	●	●	●
ATTACK	●	●	●	●	●
LOB	●	●	●	●	●
LOB DEFENSE	●	●	●	●	●
CONSISTENCY	●	●	●	●	●

KEY: **1** Not Present **2** Needs Development **3** OK **4** Good **5** Great

OBSERVE & ANALYZE

	Never	Less Often	Often	Always
Do you move the opponent to the side?				
Do you move the opponent back and forth?				
Do you give yourself enough time to get to the kitchen line when you return the serve?				
Do you demonstrate a variety of serves?				
Do you select shots appropriately?				
Do you hit into open areas of the court?				
Do you try to attack the ball at the first available opportunity?				
Do you play to the opposition's weakness?				
Do you control the point?				

What are my strengths in the gameplay areas listed above?

What are my weaknesses in the gameplay areas listed above?

How can I improve on my strengths and weaknesses in the gameplay areas listed above?

PICKLEBALL TRAINING

- [ ] Warm up/Dynamic stretching
- [ ] Cardio
- [ ] Strength training
- [ ] Drills
- [ ] Recreational play
- [ ] Semi-competitive play
- [ ] Competitive play
- [ ] Tournament play
- [ ] Cool down/Static stretching

NOTES

LONG-TERM GOALS

PICKLEBALL PLANNER

Month _____ Week _____

Date _____
Location _____
Players _____
_____
Scores _____ _____ _____

Date _____
Location _____
Players _____
_____
Scores _____ _____ _____

Date _____
Location _____
Players _____
_____
Scores _____ _____ _____

Date _____
Location _____
Players _____
_____
Scores _____ _____ _____

Date _____
Location _____
Players _____
_____
Scores _____ _____ _____

Date _____
Location _____
Players _____
_____
Scores _____ _____ _____

Date _____
Location _____
Players _____
_____
Scores _____ _____ _____

Date _____
Location _____
Players _____
_____
Scores _____ _____ _____

Things to improve on:

Player notes:

PICKLEBALL PLANNER

Month _____ Week _____

Date _____
Location _____
Players _____
_____
Scores _____ _____ _____

Date _____
Location _____
Players _____
_____
Scores _____ _____ _____

Date _____
Location _____
Players _____
_____
Scores _____ _____ _____

Date _____
Location _____
Players _____
_____
Scores _____ _____ _____

Date _____
Location _____
Players _____
_____
Scores _____ _____ _____

Date _____
Location _____
Players _____
_____
Scores _____ _____ _____

Date _____
Location _____
Players _____
_____
Scores _____ _____ _____

Date _____
Location _____
Players _____
_____
Scores _____ _____ _____

Things to improve on:

Player notes:

PICKLEBALL PLANNER

Month _____ **Week** _____

Date _____
Location _____
Players _____
_____
Scores _____ _____ _____

Date _____
Location _____
Players _____
_____
Scores _____ _____ _____

Date _____
Location _____
Players _____
_____
Scores _____ _____ _____

Date _____
Location _____
Players _____
_____
Scores _____ _____ _____

Date _____
Location _____
Players _____
_____
Scores _____ _____ _____

Date _____
Location _____
Players _____
_____
Scores _____ _____ _____

Date _____
Location _____
Players _____
_____
Scores _____ _____ _____

Date _____
Location _____
Players _____
_____
Scores _____ _____ _____

Things to improve on:

Player notes:

PICKLEBALL PLANNER

Month _____ Week _____

Date _____
Location _____
Players _____
_____
Scores _____ _____ _____

Date _____
Location _____
Players _____
_____
Scores _____ _____ _____

Date _____
Location _____
Players _____
_____
Scores _____ _____ _____

Date _____
Location _____
Players _____
_____
Scores _____ _____ _____

Date _____
Location _____
Players _____
_____
Scores _____ _____ _____

Date _____
Location _____
Players _____
_____
Scores _____ _____ _____

Date _____
Location _____
Players _____
_____
Scores _____ _____ _____

Date _____
Location _____
Players _____
_____
Scores _____ _____ _____

Things to improve on:

Player notes:

SKILLS ASSESSMENT

SKILLS	1	2	3	4	5
SERVE					
RETURN					
3RD SHOT DRIVE					
TRANSITION ZONE					
DIGS					
BLOCKING					
DINKING					
VOLLEYS					
ATTACK					
LOB					
LOB DEFENSE					
CONSISTENCY					

KEY: **1** Not Present   **2** Needs Development   **3** OK   **4** Good   **5** Great

OBSERVE & ANALYZE

	Never	Less Often	Often	Always
Do you move the opponent to the side?				
Do you move the opponent back and forth?				
Do you give yourself enough time to get to the kitchen line when you return the serve?				
Do you demonstrate a variety of serves?				
Do you select shots appropriately?				
Do you hit into open areas of the court?				
Do you try to attack the ball at the first available opportunity?				
Do you play to the opposition's weakness?				
Do you control the point?				

What are my strengths in the gameplay areas listed above?

What are my weaknesses in the gameplay areas listed above?

How can I improve on my strengths and weaknesses in the gameplay areas listed above?

PICKLEBALL TRAINING

- [ ] Warm up/Dynamic stretching
- [ ] Cardio
- [ ] Strength training
- [ ] Drills
- [ ] Recreational play
- [ ] Semi-competitive play
- [ ] Competitive play
- [ ] Tournament play
- [ ] Cool down/Static stretching

NOTES

LONG-TERM GOALS

PICKLEBALL PLANNER

Month _____ Week _____

Date _____
Location _____
Players _____
_____
Scores _____ _____ _____

Date _____
Location _____
Players _____
_____
Scores _____ _____ _____

Date _____
Location _____
Players _____
_____
Scores _____ _____ _____

Date _____
Location _____
Players _____
_____
Scores _____ _____ _____

Date _____
Location _____
Players _____
_____
Scores _____ _____ _____

Date _____
Location _____
Players _____
_____
Scores _____ _____ _____

Date _____
Location _____
Players _____
_____
Scores _____ _____ _____

Date _____
Location _____
Players _____
_____
Scores _____ _____ _____

Things to improve on:

Player notes:

PICKLEBALL PLANNER

Month _____ Week _____

Date _____
Location _____
Players _____
_____
Scores _____ _____ _____

Date _____
Location _____
Players _____
_____
Scores _____ _____ _____

Date _____
Location _____
Players _____
_____
Scores _____ _____ _____

Date _____
Location _____
Players _____
_____
Scores _____ _____ _____

Date _____
Location _____
Players _____
_____
Scores _____ _____ _____

Date _____
Location _____
Players _____
_____
Scores _____ _____ _____

Date _____
Location _____
Players _____
_____
Scores _____ _____ _____

Date _____
Location _____
Players _____
_____
Scores _____ _____ _____

Things to improve on:

Player notes:

PICKLEBALL PLANNER

Month _____   Week _____

Date _____
Location _____
Players _____
_____
Scores _____ _____ _____

Date _____
Location _____
Players _____
_____
Scores _____ _____ _____

Date _____
Location _____
Players _____
_____
Scores _____ _____ _____

Date _____
Location _____
Players _____
_____
Scores _____ _____ _____

Date _____
Location _____
Players _____
_____
Scores _____ _____ _____

Date _____
Location _____
Players _____
_____
Scores _____ _____ _____

Date _____
Location _____
Players _____
_____
Scores _____ _____ _____

Date _____
Location _____
Players _____
_____
Scores _____ _____ _____

Things to improve on:

Player notes:

PICKLEBALL PLANNER

Month _____ **Week** _____

Date _____
Location _____
Players _____
_____
Scores _____ _____ _____

Date _____
Location _____
Players _____
_____
Scores _____ _____ _____

Date _____
Location _____
Players _____
_____
Scores _____ _____ _____

Date _____
Location _____
Players _____
_____
Scores _____ _____ _____

Date _____
Location _____
Players _____
_____
Scores _____ _____ _____

Date _____
Location _____
Players _____
_____
Scores _____ _____ _____

Date _____
Location _____
Players _____
_____
Scores _____ _____ _____

Date _____
Location _____
Players _____
_____
Scores _____ _____ _____

Things to improve on:

Player notes:

SKILLS ASSESSMENT

SKILLS	1	2	3	4	5
SERVE					
RETURN					
3RD SHOT DRIVE					
TRANSITION ZONE					
DIGS					
BLOCKING					
DINKING					
VOLLEYS					
ATTACK					
LOB					
LOB DEFENSE					
CONSISTENCY					

KEY: **1** Not Present **2** Needs Development **3** OK **4** Good **5** Great

OBSERVE & ANALYZE

	Never	Less Often	Often	Always
Do you move the opponent to the side?				
Do you move the opponent back and forth?				
Do you give yourself enough time to get to the kitchen line when you return the serve?				
Do you demonstrate a variety of serves?				
Do you select shots appropriately?				
Do you hit into open areas of the court?				
Do you try to attack the ball at the first available opportunity?				
Do you play to the opposition's weakness?				
Do you control the point?				

What are my strengths in the gameplay areas listed above?

What are my weaknesses in the gameplay areas listed above?

How can I improve on my strengths and weaknesses in the gameplay areas listed above?

PICKLEBALL TRAINING

- [ ] Warm up/Dynamic stretching
- [ ] Cardio
- [ ] Strength training
- [ ] Drills
- [ ] Recreational play
- [ ] Semi-competitive play
- [ ] Competitive play
- [ ] Tournament play
- [ ] Cool down/Static stretching

NOTES

LONG-TERM GOALS

PICKLEBALL PLANNER

Month _____ **Week** _____

Date _____
Location _____
Players _____
_____
Scores _____ _____ _____

Date _____
Location _____
Players _____
_____
Scores _____ _____ _____

Date _____
Location _____
Players _____
_____
Scores _____ _____ _____

Date _____
Location _____
Players _____
_____
Scores _____ _____ _____

Date _____
Location _____
Players _____
_____
Scores _____ _____ _____

Date _____
Location _____
Players _____
_____
Scores _____ _____ _____

Date _____
Location _____
Players _____
_____
Scores _____ _____ _____

Date _____
Location _____
Players _____
_____
Scores _____ _____ _____

Things to improve on:

Player notes:

PICKLEBALL PLANNER

Month _____ Week _____

Date _____
Location _____
Players _____
_____
Scores _____ _____ _____

Date _____
Location _____
Players _____
_____
Scores _____ _____ _____

Date _____
Location _____
Players _____
_____
Scores _____ _____ _____

Date _____
Location _____
Players _____
_____
Scores _____ _____ _____

Date _____
Location _____
Players _____
_____
Scores _____ _____ _____

Date _____
Location _____
Players _____
_____
Scores _____ _____ _____

Date _____
Location _____
Players _____
_____
Scores _____ _____ _____

Date _____
Location _____
Players _____
_____
Scores _____ _____ _____

Things to improve on:

Player notes:

PICKLEBALL PLANNER

Month _____ **Week** _____

Date _____
Location _____
Players _____
_____
Scores _____ _____ _____

Date _____
Location _____
Players _____
_____
Scores _____ _____ _____

Date _____
Location _____
Players _____
_____
Scores _____ _____ _____

Date _____
Location _____
Players _____
_____
Scores _____ _____ _____

Date _____
Location _____
Players _____
_____
Scores _____ _____ _____

Date _____
Location _____
Players _____
_____
Scores _____ _____ _____

Date _____
Location _____
Players _____
_____
Scores _____ _____ _____

Date _____
Location _____
Players _____
_____
Scores _____ _____ _____

Things to improve on:

Player notes:

PICKLEBALL PLANNER

Month _____ Week _____

Date _____
Location _____
Players _____
_____
Scores _____ _____ _____

Date _____
Location _____
Players _____
_____
Scores _____ _____ _____

Date _____
Location _____
Players _____
_____
Scores _____ _____ _____

Date _____
Location _____
Players _____
_____
Scores _____ _____ _____

Date _____
Location _____
Players _____
_____
Scores _____ _____ _____

Date _____
Location _____
Players _____
_____
Scores _____ _____ _____

Date _____
Location _____
Players _____
_____
Scores _____ _____ _____

Date _____
Location _____
Players _____
_____
Scores _____ _____ _____

Things to improve on:

Player notes:

SKILLS ASSESSMENT

SKILLS	1	2	3	4	5
SERVE					
RETURN					
3RD SHOT DRIVE					
TRANSITION ZONE					
DIGS					
BLOCKING					
DINKING					
VOLLEYS					
ATTACK					
LOB					
LOB DEFENSE					
CONSISTENCY					

KEY: **1** Not Present   **2** Needs Development   **3** OK   **4** Good   **5** Great

OBSERVE & ANALYZE

	Never	Less Often	Often	Always
Do you move the opponent to the side?				
Do you move the opponent back and forth?				
Do you give yourself enough time to get to the kitchen line when you return the serve?				
Do you demonstrate a variety of serves?				
Do you select shots appropriately?				
Do you hit into open areas of the court?				
Do you try to attack the ball at the first available opportunity?				
Do you play to the opposition's weakness?				
Do you control the point?				

What are my strengths in the gameplay areas listed above?

What are my weaknesses in the gameplay areas listed above?

How can I improve on my strengths and weaknesses in the gameplay areas listed above?

PICKLEBALL TRAINING

- ☐ Warm up/Dynamic stretching
- ☐ Cardio
- ☐ Strength training
- ☐ Drills
- ☐ Recreational play
- ☐ Semi-competitive play
- ☐ Competitive play
- ☐ Tournament play
- ☐ Cool down/Static stretching

NOTES

LONG-TERM GOALS

- [ ]
- [ ]
- [ ]
- [ ]
- [ ]
- [ ]
- [ ]
- [ ]
- [ ]
- [ ]
- [ ]
- [ ]
- [ ]
- [ ]
- [ ]
- [ ]
- [ ]
- [ ]
- [ ]
- [ ]
- [ ]
- [ ]

PICKLEBALL PLANNER

Month _____ Week _____

Date _____
Location _____
Players _____
_____
Scores _____ _____ _____

Date _____
Location _____
Players _____
_____
Scores _____ _____ _____

Date _____
Location _____
Players _____
_____
Scores _____ _____ _____

Date _____
Location _____
Players _____
_____
Scores _____ _____ _____

Date _____
Location _____
Players _____
_____
Scores _____ _____ _____

Date _____
Location _____
Players _____
_____
Scores _____ _____ _____

Date _____
Location _____
Players _____
_____
Scores _____ _____ _____

Date _____
Location _____
Players _____
_____
Scores _____ _____ _____

Things to improve on:

Player notes:

PICKLEBALL PLANNER

Month _____ Week _____

Date _____
Location _____
Players _____
_____
Scores _____ _____ _____

Date _____
Location _____
Players _____
_____
Scores _____ _____ _____

Date _____
Location _____
Players _____
_____
Scores _____ _____ _____

Date _____
Location _____
Players _____
_____
Scores _____ _____ _____

Date _____
Location _____
Players _____
_____
Scores _____ _____ _____

Date _____
Location _____
Players _____
_____
Scores _____ _____ _____

Date _____
Location _____
Players _____
_____
Scores _____ _____ _____

Date _____
Location _____
Players _____
_____
Scores _____ _____ _____

Things to improve on:

Player notes:

PICKLEBALL PLANNER

Month _____ **Week** _____

Date _____
Location _____
Players _____
_____
Scores _____ _____ _____

Date _____
Location _____
Players _____
_____
Scores _____ _____ _____

Date _____
Location _____
Players _____
_____
Scores _____ _____ _____

Date _____
Location _____
Players _____
_____
Scores _____ _____ _____

Date _____
Location _____
Players _____
_____
Scores _____ _____ _____

Date _____
Location _____
Players _____
_____
Scores _____ _____ _____

Date _____
Location _____
Players _____
_____
Scores _____ _____ _____

Date _____
Location _____
Players _____
_____
Scores _____ _____ _____

Things to improve on:

Player notes:

PICKLEBALL PLANNER

Month _____ Week _____

Date _____
Location _____
Players _____
_____
Scores _____ _____ _____

Date _____
Location _____
Players _____
_____
Scores _____ _____ _____

Date _____
Location _____
Players _____
_____
Scores _____ _____ _____

Date _____
Location _____
Players _____
_____
Scores _____ _____ _____

Date _____
Location _____
Players _____
_____
Scores _____ _____ _____

Date _____
Location _____
Players _____
_____
Scores _____ _____ _____

Date _____
Location _____
Players _____
_____
Scores _____ _____ _____

Date _____
Location _____
Players _____
_____
Scores _____ _____ _____

Things to improve on:

Player notes:

SKILLS ASSESSMENT

SKILLS	1	2	3	4	5
SERVE					
RETURN					
3RD SHOT DRIVE					
TRANSITION ZONE					
DIGS					
BLOCKING					
DINKING					
VOLLEYS					
ATTACK					
LOB					
LOB DEFENSE					
CONSISTENCY					

KEY: **1** Not Present   **2** Needs Development   **3** OK   **4** Good   **5** Great

OBSERVE & ANALYZE

	Never	Less Often	Often	Always
Do you move the opponent to the side?				
Do you move the opponent back and forth?				
Do you give yourself enough time to get to the kitchen line when you return the serve?				
Do you demonstrate a variety of serves?				
Do you select shots appropriately?				
Do you hit into open areas of the court?				
Do you try to attack the ball at the first available opportunity?				
Do you play to the opposition's weakness?				
Do you control the point?				

What are my strengths in the gameplay areas listed above?

What are my weaknesses in the gameplay areas listed above?

How can I improve on my strengths and weaknesses in the gameplay areas listed above?

PICKLEBALL TRAINING

- [ ] Warm up/Dynamic stretching
- [ ] Cardio
- [ ] Strength training
- [ ] Drills
- [ ] Recreational play
- [ ] Semi-competitive play
- [ ] Competitive play
- [ ] Tournament play
- [ ] Cool down/Static stretching

NOTES

LONG-TERM GOALS

PICKLEBALL PLANNER

Month _____ **Week** _____

Date _____
Location _____
Players _____
_____
Scores _____ _____ _____

Date _____
Location _____
Players _____
_____
Scores _____ _____ _____

Date _____
Location _____
Players _____
_____
Scores _____ _____ _____

Date _____
Location _____
Players _____
_____
Scores _____ _____ _____

Date _____
Location _____
Players _____
_____
Scores _____ _____ _____

Date _____
Location _____
Players _____
_____
Scores _____ _____ _____

Date _____
Location _____
Players _____
_____
Scores _____ _____ _____

Date _____
Location _____
Players _____
_____
Scores _____ _____ _____

Things to improve on:

Player notes:

PICKLEBALL PLANNER

Month _____ Week _____

Date _____
Location _____
Players _____
_____
Scores _____ _____ _____

Date _____
Location _____
Players _____
_____
Scores _____ _____ _____

Date _____
Location _____
Players _____
_____
Scores _____ _____ _____

Date _____
Location _____
Players _____
_____
Scores _____ _____ _____

Date _____
Location _____
Players _____
_____
Scores _____ _____ _____

Date _____
Location _____
Players _____
_____
Scores _____ _____ _____

Date _____
Location _____
Players _____
_____
Scores _____ _____ _____

Date _____
Location _____
Players _____
_____
Scores _____ _____ _____

Things to improve on:

Player notes:

PICKLEBALL PLANNER

Month _____ **Week** _____

Date _____
Location _____
Players _____
_____
Scores _____ _____ _____

Date _____
Location _____
Players _____
_____
Scores _____ _____ _____

Date _____
Location _____
Players _____
_____
Scores _____ _____ _____

Date _____
Location _____
Players _____
_____
Scores _____ _____ _____

Date _____
Location _____
Players _____
_____
Scores _____ _____ _____

Date _____
Location _____
Players _____
_____
Scores _____ _____ _____

Date _____
Location _____
Players _____
_____
Scores _____ _____ _____

Date _____
Location _____
Players _____
_____
Scores _____ _____ _____

Things to improve on:

Player notes:

PICKLEBALL PLANNER

Month _____ Week _____

Date _____
Location _____
Players _____
_____
Scores _____ _____ _____

Date _____
Location _____
Players _____
_____
Scores _____ _____ _____

Date _____
Location _____
Players _____
_____
Scores _____ _____ _____

Date _____
Location _____
Players _____
_____
Scores _____ _____ _____

Date _____
Location _____
Players _____
_____
Scores _____ _____ _____

Date _____
Location _____
Players _____
_____
Scores _____ _____ _____

Date _____
Location _____
Players _____
_____
Scores _____ _____ _____

Date _____
Location _____
Players _____
_____
Scores _____ _____ _____

Things to improve on:

Player notes:

SKILLS ASSESSMENT

SKILLS	1	2	3	4	5
SERVE					
RETURN					
3RD SHOT DRIVE					
TRANSITION ZONE					
DIGS					
BLOCKING					
DINKING					
VOLLEYS					
ATTACK					
LOB					
LOB DEFENSE					
CONSISTENCY					

KEY: **1** Not Present   **2** Needs Development   **3** OK   **4** Good   **5** Great

OBSERVE & ANALYZE

	Never	Less Often	Often	Always
Do you move the opponent to the side?				
Do you move the opponent back and forth?				
Do you give yourself enough time to get to the kitchen line when you return the serve?				
Do you demonstrate a variety of serves?				
Do you select shots appropriately?				
Do you hit into open areas of the court?				
Do you try to attack the ball at the first available opportunity?				
Do you play to the opposition's weakness?				
Do you control the point?				

What are my strengths in the gameplay areas listed above?

What are my weaknesses in the gameplay areas listed above?

How can I improve on my strengths and weaknesses in the gameplay areas listed above?

PICKLEBALL TRAINING

- [ ] Warm up/Dynamic stretching
- [ ] Cardio
- [ ] Strength training
- [ ] Drills
- [ ] Recreational play
- [ ] Semi-competitive play
- [ ] Competitive play
- [ ] Tournament play
- [ ] Cool down/Static stretching

NOTES

LONG-TERM GOALS

PICKLEBALL PLANNER

Month _____ **Week** _____

Date _____
Location _____
Players _____
_____
Scores _____ _____ _____

Date _____
Location _____
Players _____
_____
Scores _____ _____ _____

Date _____
Location _____
Players _____
_____
Scores _____ _____ _____

Date _____
Location _____
Players _____
_____
Scores _____ _____ _____

Date _____
Location _____
Players _____
_____
Scores _____ _____ _____

Date _____
Location _____
Players _____
_____
Scores _____ _____ _____

Date _____
Location _____
Players _____
_____
Scores _____ _____ _____

Date _____
Location _____
Players _____
_____
Scores _____ _____ _____

Things to improve on:

Player notes:

PICKLEBALL PLANNER

Month _____ Week _____

Date _____
Location _____
Players _____
_____
Scores _____ _____ _____

Date _____
Location _____
Players _____
_____
Scores _____ _____ _____

Date _____
Location _____
Players _____
_____
Scores _____ _____ _____

Date _____
Location _____
Players _____
_____
Scores _____ _____ _____

Date _____
Location _____
Players _____
_____
Scores _____ _____ _____

Date _____
Location _____
Players _____
_____
Scores _____ _____ _____

Date _____
Location _____
Players _____
_____
Scores _____ _____ _____

Date _____
Location _____
Players _____
_____
Scores _____ _____ _____

Things to improve on:

Player notes:

PICKLEBALL PLANNER

Month _____ **Week** _____

Date _____
Location _____
Players _____
_____
Scores _____ _____ _____

Date _____
Location _____
Players _____
_____
Scores _____ _____ _____

Date _____
Location _____
Players _____
_____
Scores _____ _____ _____

Date _____
Location _____
Players _____
_____
Scores _____ _____ _____

Date _____
Location _____
Players _____
_____
Scores _____ _____ _____

Date _____
Location _____
Players _____
_____
Scores _____ _____ _____

Date _____
Location _____
Players _____
_____
Scores _____ _____ _____

Date _____
Location _____
Players _____
_____
Scores _____ _____ _____

Things to improve on:

Player notes:

PICKLEBALL PLANNER

Month _____ **Week** _____

Date _____
Location _____
Players _____
_____
Scores _____ _____ _____

Date _____
Location _____
Players _____
_____
Scores _____ _____ _____

Date _____
Location _____
Players _____
_____
Scores _____ _____ _____

Date _____
Location _____
Players _____
_____
Scores _____ _____ _____

Date _____
Location _____
Players _____
_____
Scores _____ _____ _____

Date _____
Location _____
Players _____
_____
Scores _____ _____ _____

Date _____
Location _____
Players _____
_____
Scores _____ _____ _____

Date _____
Location _____
Players _____
_____
Scores _____ _____ _____

Things to improve on:

Player notes:

SKILLS ASSESSMENT

SKILLS	1	2	3	4	5
SERVE	○	○	○	○	○
RETURN	○	○	○	○	○
3RD SHOT DRIVE	○	○	○	○	○
TRANSITION ZONE	○	○	○	○	○
DIGS	○	○	○	○	○
BLOCKING	○	○	○	○	○
DINKING	○	○	○	○	○
VOLLEYS	○	○	○	○	○
ATTACK	○	○	○	○	○
LOB	○	○	○	○	○
LOB DEFENSE	○	○	○	○	○
CONSISTENCY	○	○	○	○	○

KEY: **1** Not Present **2** Needs Development **3** OK **4** Good **5** Great

OBSERVE & ANALYZE

	Never	Less Often	Often	Always
Do you move the opponent to the side?				
Do you move the opponent back and forth?				
Do you give yourself enough time to get to the kitchen line when you return the serve?				
Do you demonstrate a variety of serves?				
Do you select shots appropriately?				
Do you hit into open areas of the court?				
Do you try to attack the ball at the first available opportunity?				
Do you play to the opposition's weakness?				
Do you control the point?				

What are my strengths in the gameplay areas listed above?

What are my weaknesses in the gameplay areas listed above?

How can I improve on my strengths and weaknesses in the gameplay areas listed above?

PICKLEBALL TRAINING

- [ ] Warm up/Dynamic stretching
- [ ] Cardio
- [ ] Strength training
- [ ] Drills
- [ ] Recreational play
- [ ] Semi-competitive play
- [ ] Competitive play
- [ ] Tournament play
- [ ] Cool down/Static stretching

NOTES

LONG-TERM GOALS

PICKLEBALL PLANNER

Month _____ **Week** _____

Date _____
Location _____
Players _____
_____
Scores _____ _____ _____

Date _____
Location _____
Players _____
_____
Scores _____ _____ _____

Date _____
Location _____
Players _____
_____
Scores _____ _____ _____

Date _____
Location _____
Players _____
_____
Scores _____ _____ _____

Date _____
Location _____
Players _____
_____
Scores _____ _____ _____

Date _____
Location _____
Players _____
_____
Scores _____ _____ _____

Date _____
Location _____
Players _____
_____
Scores _____ _____ _____

Date _____
Location _____
Players _____
_____
Scores _____ _____ _____

Things to improve on:

Player notes:

PICKLEBALL PLANNER

Month _____ Week _____

Date _____
Location _____
Players _____
_____
Scores _____ _____ _____

Date _____
Location _____
Players _____
_____
Scores _____ _____ _____

Date _____
Location _____
Players _____
_____
Scores _____ _____ _____

Date _____
Location _____
Players _____
_____
Scores _____ _____ _____

Date _____
Location _____
Players _____
_____
Scores _____ _____ _____

Date _____
Location _____
Players _____
_____
Scores _____ _____ _____

Date _____
Location _____
Players _____
_____
Scores _____ _____ _____

Date _____
Location _____
Players _____
_____
Scores _____ _____ _____

Things to improve on:

Player notes:

PICKLEBALL PLANNER

Month _____ **Week** _____

Date _____
Location _____
Players _____
_____
Scores _____ _____ _____

Date _____
Location _____
Players _____
_____
Scores _____ _____ _____

Date _____
Location _____
Players _____
_____
Scores _____ _____ _____

Date _____
Location _____
Players _____
_____
Scores _____ _____ _____

Date _____
Location _____
Players _____
_____
Scores _____ _____ _____

Date _____
Location _____
Players _____
_____
Scores _____ _____ _____

Date _____
Location _____
Players _____
_____
Scores _____ _____ _____

Date _____
Location _____
Players _____
_____
Scores _____ _____ _____

Things to improve on:

Player notes:

PICKLEBALL PLANNER

Month _____ Week _____

Date _____
Location _____
Players _____
_____
Scores _____ _____ _____

Date _____
Location _____
Players _____
_____
Scores _____ _____ _____

Date _____
Location _____
Players _____
_____
Scores _____ _____ _____

Date _____
Location _____
Players _____
_____
Scores _____ _____ _____

Date _____
Location _____
Players _____
_____
Scores _____ _____ _____

Date _____
Location _____
Players _____
_____
Scores _____ _____ _____

Date _____
Location _____
Players _____
_____
Scores _____ _____ _____

Date _____
Location _____
Players _____
_____
Scores _____ _____ _____

Things to improve on:

Player notes:

SKILLS ASSESSMENT

SKILLS	1	2	3	4	5
SERVE					
RETURN					
3RD SHOT DRIVE					
TRANSITION ZONE					
DIGS					
BLOCKING					
DINKING					
VOLLEYS					
ATTACK					
LOB					
LOB DEFENSE					
CONSISTENCY					

KEY: **1** Not Present   **2** Needs Development   **3** OK   **4** Good   **5** Great

OBSERVE & ANALYZE

	Never	Less Often	Often	Always
Do you move the opponent to the side?				
Do you move the opponent back and forth?				
Do you give yourself enough time to get to the kitchen line when you return the serve?				
Do you demonstrate a variety of serves?				
Do you select shots appropriately?				
Do you hit into open areas of the court?				
Do you try to attack the ball at the first available opportunity?				
Do you play to the opposition's weakness?				
Do you control the point?				

What are my strengths in the gameplay areas listed above?

What are my weaknesses in the gameplay areas listed above?

How can I improve on my strengths and weaknesses in the gameplay areas listed above?

PICKLEBALL TRAINING

- [ ] Warm up/Dynamic stretching
- [ ] Cardio
- [ ] Strength training
- [ ] Drills
- [ ] Recreational play
- [ ] Semi-competitive play
- [ ] Competitive play
- [ ] Tournament play
- [ ] Cool down/Static stretching

NOTES

LONG-TERM GOALS

PICKLEBALL PLANNER

Month _____ **Week** _____

Date _____
Location _____
Players _____
_____
Scores _____ _____ _____

Date _____
Location _____
Players _____
_____
Scores _____ _____ _____

Date _____
Location _____
Players _____
_____
Scores _____ _____ _____

Date _____
Location _____
Players _____
_____
Scores _____ _____ _____

Date _____
Location _____
Players _____
_____
Scores _____ _____ _____

Date _____
Location _____
Players _____
_____
Scores _____ _____ _____

Date _____
Location _____
Players _____
_____
Scores _____ _____ _____

Date _____
Location _____
Players _____
_____
Scores _____ _____ _____

Things to improve on:

Player notes:

PICKLEBALL PLANNER

Month _____ Week _____

Date _____
Location _____
Players _____
_____
Scores _____ _____ _____

Date _____
Location _____
Players _____
_____
Scores _____ _____ _____

Date _____
Location _____
Players _____
_____
Scores _____ _____ _____

Date _____
Location _____
Players _____
_____
Scores _____ _____ _____

Date _____
Location _____
Players _____
_____
Scores _____ _____ _____

Date _____
Location _____
Players _____
_____
Scores _____ _____ _____

Date _____
Location _____
Players _____
_____
Scores _____ _____ _____

Date _____
Location _____
Players _____
_____
Scores _____ _____ _____

Things to improve on:

Player notes:

PICKLEBALL PLANNER

Month _____ **Week** _____

Date _____
Location _____
Players _____
_____
Scores _____ _____ _____

Date _____
Location _____
Players _____
_____
Scores _____ _____ _____

Date _____
Location _____
Players _____
_____
Scores _____ _____ _____

Date _____
Location _____
Players _____
_____
Scores _____ _____ _____

Date _____
Location _____
Players _____
_____
Scores _____ _____ _____

Date _____
Location _____
Players _____
_____
Scores _____ _____ _____

Date _____
Location _____
Players _____
_____
Scores _____ _____ _____

Date _____
Location _____
Players _____
_____
Scores _____ _____ _____

Things to improve on:

Player notes:

PICKLEBALL PLANNER

Month _____ Week _____

Date _____
Location _____
Players _____
_____
Scores _____ _____ _____

Date _____
Location _____
Players _____
_____
Scores _____ _____ _____

Date _____
Location _____
Players _____
_____
Scores _____ _____ _____

Date _____
Location _____
Players _____
_____
Scores _____ _____ _____

Date _____
Location _____
Players _____
_____
Scores _____ _____ _____

Date _____
Location _____
Players _____
_____
Scores _____ _____ _____

Date _____
Location _____
Players _____
_____
Scores _____ _____ _____

Date _____
Location _____
Players _____
_____
Scores _____ _____ _____

Things to improve on:

Player notes:

SKILLS ASSESSMENT

SKILLS	1	2	3	4	5
SERVE	○	○	○	○	○
RETURN	○	○	○	○	○
3RD SHOT DRIVE	○	○	○	○	○
TRANSITION ZONE	○	○	○	○	○
DIGS	○	○	○	○	○
BLOCKING	○	○	○	○	○
DINKING	○	○	○	○	○
VOLLEYS	○	○	○	○	○
ATTACK	○	○	○	○	○
LOB	○	○	○	○	○
LOB DEFENSE	○	○	○	○	○
CONSISTENCY	○	○	○	○	○

KEY: **1** Not Present   **2** Needs Development   **3** OK   **4** Good   **5** Great

OBSERVE & ANALYZE

	Never	Less Often	Often	Always
Do you move the opponent to the side?				
Do you move the opponent back and forth?				
Do you give yourself enough time to get to the kitchen line when you return the serve?				
Do you demonstrate a variety of serves?				
Do you select shots appropriately?				
Do you hit into open areas of the court?				
Do you try to attack the ball at the first available opportunity?				
Do you play to the opposition's weakness?				
Do you control the point?				

What are my strengths in the gameplay areas listed above?

What are my weaknesses in the gameplay areas listed above?

How can I improve on my strengths and weaknesses in the gameplay areas listed above?

PICKLEBALL TRAINING

- [ ] Warm up/Dynamic stretching
- [ ] Cardio
- [ ] Strength training
- [ ] Drills
- [ ] Recreational play
- [ ] Semi-competitive play
- [ ] Competitive play
- [ ] Tournament play
- [ ] Cool down/Static stretching

NOTES

LONG-TERM GOALS

PICKLEBALL PLANNER

Month _____ **Week** _____

Date _____
Location _____
Players _____
_____
Scores _____ _____ _____

Date _____
Location _____
Players _____
_____
Scores _____ _____ _____

Date _____
Location _____
Players _____
_____
Scores _____ _____ _____

Date _____
Location _____
Players _____
_____
Scores _____ _____ _____

Date _____
Location _____
Players _____
_____
Scores _____ _____ _____

Date _____
Location _____
Players _____
_____
Scores _____ _____ _____

Date _____
Location _____
Players _____
_____
Scores _____ _____ _____

Date _____
Location _____
Players _____
_____
Scores _____ _____ _____

Things to improve on:

Player notes:

PICKLEBALL PLANNER

Month _____ Week _____

Date _____
Location _____
Players _____
_____
Scores _____ _____ _____

Date _____
Location _____
Players _____
_____
Scores _____ _____ _____

Date _____
Location _____
Players _____
_____
Scores _____ _____ _____

Date _____
Location _____
Players _____
_____
Scores _____ _____ _____

Date _____
Location _____
Players _____
_____
Scores _____ _____ _____

Date _____
Location _____
Players _____
_____
Scores _____ _____ _____

Date _____
Location _____
Players _____
_____
Scores _____ _____ _____

Date _____
Location _____
Players _____
_____
Scores _____ _____ _____

Things to improve on:

Player notes:

PICKLEBALL PLANNER

Month _____ **Week** _____

Date _____
Location _____
Players _____
_____
Scores _____ _____ _____

Date _____
Location _____
Players _____
_____
Scores _____ _____ _____

Date _____
Location _____
Players _____
_____
Scores _____ _____ _____

Date _____
Location _____
Players _____
_____
Scores _____ _____ _____

Date _____
Location _____
Players _____
_____
Scores _____ _____ _____

Date _____
Location _____
Players _____
_____
Scores _____ _____ _____

Date _____
Location _____
Players _____
_____
Scores _____ _____ _____

Date _____
Location _____
Players _____
_____
Scores _____ _____ _____

Things to improve on:

Player notes:

PICKLEBALL PLANNER

Month _____ Week _____

Date _____
Location _____
Players _____
_____
Scores _____ _____ _____

Date _____
Location _____
Players _____
_____
Scores _____ _____ _____

Date _____
Location _____
Players _____
_____
Scores _____ _____ _____

Date _____
Location _____
Players _____
_____
Scores _____ _____ _____

Date _____
Location _____
Players _____
_____
Scores _____ _____ _____

Date _____
Location _____
Players _____
_____
Scores _____ _____ _____

Date _____
Location _____
Players _____
_____
Scores _____ _____ _____

Date _____
Location _____
Players _____
_____
Scores _____ _____ _____

Things to improve on:

Player notes:

SKILLS ASSESSMENT

SKILLS	1	2	3	4	5
SERVE					
RETURN					
3RD SHOT DRIVE					
TRANSITION ZONE					
DIGS					
BLOCKING					
DINKING					
VOLLEYS					
ATTACK					
LOB					
LOB DEFENSE					
CONSISTENCY					

KEY: **1** Not Present   **2** Needs Development   **3** OK   **4** Good   **5** Great

OBSERVE & ANALYZE

	Never	Less Often	Often	Always
Do you move the opponent to the side?				
Do you move the opponent back and forth?				
Do you give yourself enough time to get to the kitchen line when you return the serve?				
Do you demonstrate a variety of serves?				
Do you select shots appropriately?				
Do you hit into open areas of the court?				
Do you try to attack the ball at the first available opportunity?				
Do you play to the opposition's weakness?				
Do you control the point?				

What are my strengths in the gameplay areas listed above?

What are my weaknesses in the gameplay areas listed above?

How can I improve on my strengths and weaknesses in the gameplay areas listed above?

PICKLEBALL TRAINING

- [ ] Warm up/Dynamic stretching
- [ ] Cardio
- [ ] Strength training
- [ ] Drills
- [ ] Recreational play
- [ ] Semi-competitive play
- [ ] Competitive play
- [ ] Tournament play
- [ ] Cool down/Static stretching

NOTES

LONG-TERM GOALS

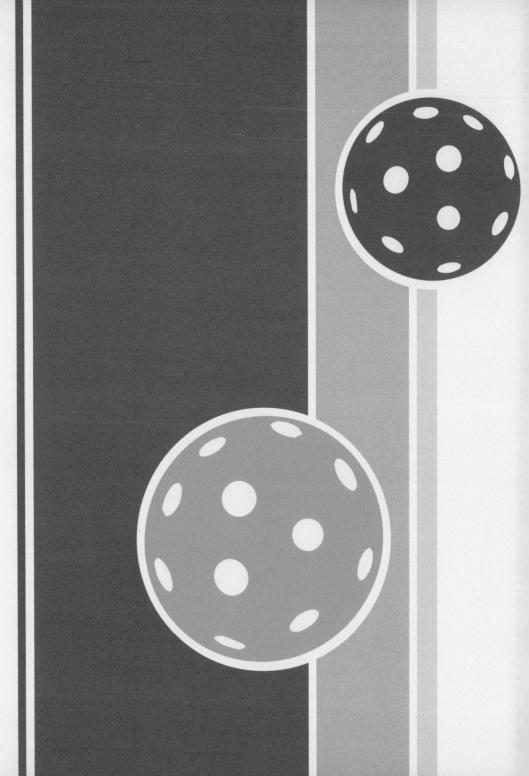

ABOUT THE AUTHOR

Sydney Steinaker is a social media influencer who is obsessed with a sport played with a plastic Wiffle ball and paddle. She travels all over the US and the world to play pickleball. Prior to playing pickleball, Sydney graduated from the University of California, Irvine, with a B.S. in Business Economics. She worked in law for several years before becoming an information security analyst. You can follow her on Instagram (@sydneysteinaker) and TikTok (@sydneysteinaker), and get all the latest updates on her pickleball journey via her podcast, *The Basic Dink*.

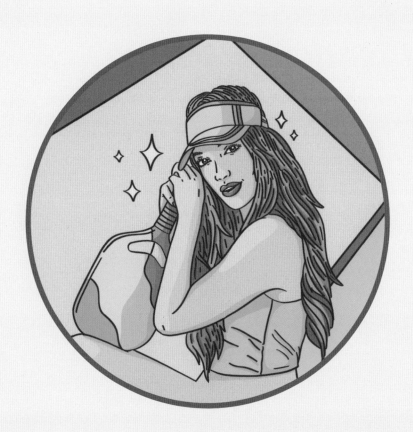

© 2023, 2024 by Quarto Publishing Group USA Inc.
Text © 2023 by Sydney Steinaker

First published in 2024 by Rock Point,
an imprint of The Quarto Group,
142 West 36th Street, 4th Floor,
New York, NY 10018, USA
(212) 779-4972
www.Quarto.com

Contains content previously published in 2023 as *Play Pickleball* by Rock Point, an imprint
of The Quarto Group, 142 West 36th Street, 4th Floor, New York, NY 10018, USA

Rock Point titles are also available at discount for retail, wholesale, promotional, and bulk
purchase. For details, contact the Special Sales Manager by email at specialsales@quarto.
com or by mail at The Quarto Group, Attn: Special Sales Manager, 100 Cummings Center
Suite 265D, Beverly, MA 01915 USA.

10 9 8 7 6 5 4 3 2 1

ISBN: 978-1-57715-450-1

Group Publisher: Rage Kindelsperger
Editorial Director: Erin Canning
Creative Director: Laura Drew
Managing Editor: Cara Donaldson
Cover Design: Scott Richardson
Illustrations: Lucía Gómez Alcaide (Lucía Types)

Printed in China